Cùnshàng Zōngzhàn's
(Jp: Sōsen Murakami)

骨度正誤

Correcting Errors in Standard Bone Measurement

Gǔ Dù Zhèng Wù
(Jp: Kotsu Do Sei Go Zu Setsu)

Dr. Yue Lu, L.Ac., Dipl.Ac.

The Chinese Medicine Database
www.cm-db.com
Portland, Oregon

Correcting Errors in Standard Bone Measurement

骨度正誤

Gǔ Dù Zhèng Wù
(Jp: Kotsu Do Sei Go Zu Setsu)

Yue Lu

Copyright © 2019 The Chinese Medicine Database

1017 SW Morrison #307A
Portland, OR 97205 USA

COMP designation original Japanese work and English translation

Cover Design by Jonathan Schell L.Ac.
Library of Congress Cataloging-in-Publication Data:

Cùnshàng Zōngzhàn (Jp: Sōsen Murakami), fl. - 1744
　　[Correcting Errors in Standard Bone Measurement. English]
　　Gu Du Zheng Wu (Jp: Kotsu Do Sei Go Zu Setsu) = Correcting Errors
in Standard Bone Measurement./ translation Yue Lu, edit Lorraine
Wilcox
　　　　p. cm.
　　Includes Index.
　　ISBN 978-0-9906029-6-5 (alk. paper)
　　Medicine, Japanese.　　　I. Lu, Yue. II. Title: Correcting Errors in
Standard Bone Measurement.

International Standard Book Number (ISBN): 978-0-9906029-6-5
Printed in the United States of America

Contents

In the original document, no page numbers are listed, simply a title for each section. However, when one turns to these sections, there is often no title or a different title, although the content matches what is given here.

Illustrations

There are two sets of point illustrations, the fiirst set has the original characters and the second set has the Western numbering system. The second set is denoted with ( )'s.

Appendices

Indices

《骨度正誤》
Introduction to *Gǔ Dù Zhèng Wù*[1]

Gǔ Dù Zhèng Wù 《骨度正誤》 (Jp: *Kotsu Do Sei Go Zu Setsu*) (Correcting Errors of Standard Bone Measurement) was written by Cùnshàng Zōngzhàn 村上宗占 (Jp: Sōsen Murakami) in 1744, during the reign of Yánxiǎng (En Kyō).

Unfortunately, no detailed information is currently available about this author. Throughout the twenty chapters in the book, the author expressed his own opinion and understanding of standard bone measurement and straw measurement which were discussed in *Huáng Dì Nèi Jīng* 《黃帝內經》 (The Yellow Emperor's Inner Classic); he also criticized Zhāng Jièbīn 張介賓 (1563–1640), a famous *Míng* dynasty doctor, about mistakes which Master Zhāng made on these same topics.

Chapter 1 provides corrected pictures and general diagrams of the channels and points from the Bronze Man (Tóng Rén) figure. In this chapter, Master Sōsen summarized the location of points in different areas of the body. He also listed points that are contraindicated for acupuncture and moxibustion.

In Chapters 2 through 14, Master Sōsen discussed standard bone measurement of the body, included measurements on the chest, abdomen, upper extremity and Dū meridian. The location of the back-transport points is also mentioned. In addition, Master Sōsen pointed out discrepancies in Master Zhāng's interpretation of certain bone measurements in *Nèi Jīng*.

In Chapter 15 through Chapter 20, Master Sōsen presented his opinion on straw or string measurement as described in *Nèi Jīng*. Diagrams were also provided to enhance the understanding of the theory.

---

1. This text was originally published by 日本橋（ エ ド ）：須原屋平左衛門 ニホンバシ（ エ ド ）：スハラヤヘイザエモン *nihonbashi(edo): suharaya-heizaemon.*

Overall, in this book, Master Sōsen challenged Zhāng Jiebīn on the theory of bone measurement and straw measurement so his thoughts give a different view for later generations and practitioners today.

Acknowledgements

I would like to express my appreciation to Lorraine Wilcox. I thank her for encouraging my work. Her comments and suggestions on the translation have been priceless. Without her help, this book would not have been possible.

A special thanks also goes to Jonathan Schell for introducing this ancient Japanese classic to the English-speaking world.

Finally, I would like to express appreciation to my family. Your support is what has sustained me thus far and given me incentive to work towards my goal.

骨度正誤

Gǔ Dù Zhèng Wù

Correcting Errors in Standard Bone Measurement

骨度正誤序

Preface for *Correcting Errors in Standard Bone Measurement*

蓋醫之術大也，人之死生系焉。而其疾病多端詳，察其癥以為之治，或藥餌，或針砭，或灸艾，或按摩，各通其一科，用以取驗。此之謂醫也。

The skill of the doctor is important; it relates to the life and death of people. There is a lot of detailed information about the diseases. [A doctor] must observe the symptoms to make decisions on treatment, either with herbs, or acupuncture and *biān* (stone needling), or moxibustion, or massage. [A doctor] who is proficient in one [of the above] specialties can use it to get the expected results. This is called a doctor.

國家升平百有余年，豪杰并起，夫人專門，不乏其術，唯經絡骨度惟難嚮。水野壹列公出村上宗占所著書示不佞，且命序，不佞熟讀其書，錯綜諸說，參考百家，正其違，刊其謬，間加己意，以發千載不言之妙。

The nation has been through over a hundred years of peace and prosperity; heroes all gather together and people specialize in [different] fields. Only the channels and network vessels, and their standard bone measurement are difficult to echo. Master Shuǐyě Yīlìe[1] showed me the book written by Cùnshàng Zōngzhàn[2] and asked me to write a preface. I read his book thoroughly; he synthesized different theories, consulted with hundreds of scholars, corrected the violations, deleted the fallacies, and occasionally added his own opinions. He expressed the mysteries that have not been spoken of for over a thousand years.

---

1. Shuǐyě Yīlìe 水野壹列 Mizuno, Ichirei: No information is currently available about this person.
2. Cùnshàng Zōngzhàn 村上宗占 or Murakami, Sōsen in Japanese, is the author of this book.

於是乎經絡之理，骨度之法，瞭然明於今。不佞箕裘之業，
自結髮時，講求經絡骨度，嘗有大疑，於是書乎，大疑頓
解。嗚呼，宗占之術可謂勤矣！別有二火一得評其言，亦可
觀也。水野公，寬宏君子，宗占屢游公門，則宗占之為人亦
可知也。不佞雖未知宗占，是以序云

Thus, the theories of the channels and network vessels, as well as the standard
bone measurement methods have now become clear. I have taken up my fa-
ther's profession since my hair was knotted up [became an adult], and have had
many questions when talking about the channels and network vessels, as well
as standard bone measurement. Those questions were resolved immediately by
this book. Sigh! The work of Zōngzhàn was helpful! It also can be found in the
evaluation of Èrhuǒ Yīdé.[3] Master Shuǐyě is a generous gentleman; Zōngzhàn
visited his house frequently, so the behavior of Zōngzhàn could also be known.
Even though I never met Zōngzhàn, I wrote this preface.

延享二歲次乙丑臘月江都官醫井上雅貴撰

In the twelfth lunar month of the *yǐ chǒu* year, the second year of Yánxiǎng's
reign (1745), written in Jiāngdū[4] by Jǐngshàng Yǎguì,[5] official doctor

---

3. Èrhuǒ Yīdé 二火一得 Ni Ka, Ittoku: No information is currently available
about this person.
4. Jiāng Dū 江都 Kō To is a nickname for Edo. Edo (えど), also Romanized as
Jedo, Yedo or Yeddo, is the former name of Tokyo.
5. Jǐngshàng Yǎguì 井上雅貴 Inoue, Masataka: No information is currently
available about this person.

骨度正誤自序

Author's Preface for Correcting Errors in Standard Bone Measurement

夫氣血者，譬如流水也。經絡者，猶堤防之在河水也。是以
流水為物，妨礙則妄行汎（泛）濫，以遂失其性也矣。人之
經絡為邪壅塞，則氣血為之不行，而疾病立至焉。欲治之
者，能視其通塞，因其正道而考其經絡，究其俞穴。於斯
也，針灸湯液施其宜，豈可不九折相慎乎？故伯仁曰：不明
經絡，則不知邪之所在，信哉此言也。

Qì and blood flow like water. Channels and network vessels are like the embankment alongside a river. Therefore, flowing water is a substance; if it is obstructed, it will flow abnormally, flooding and losing its nature. If the channels and network vessels in a human being are blocked by evils, qì and blood will be unable to flow; thus, diseases will immediately arise. People who offer treatment should be able to observe the clear or the blocked, follow the proper pathways to examine the channels and investigate the points. In this way, acupuncture or decoctions can be applied appropriately. How can we fail to practice diligently and be very careful regarding this? So Huá Bórén[6] said: If one fails to understand the channels and network vessels, one cannot know where evils will be found. These words are worthy of belief!

今也考究經絡俞穴者，或有焉，或無焉，奚得其真乎？蓋俞
穴之正道在骨度，骨度一差，則穴處無不差；而穴處差，則
灸刺非徒無益且施害於人也必矣。故聖人立骨度之法，以垂
教於後世，實不易之法也。向來經絡之書，灸刺之法，積為
卷數，周行於世，家喻戶曉，其有功於學者亦不少焉，然未
合經旨者間在矣。

---

6. Huá Bórén 滑伯仁 (1304~1386) was a famous doctor of the *Yuán* dynasty.

Nowadays, perhaps there may be people who study the channels and network vessels as well as the points, but do they get the true meaning? The correct way of [locating] points is in standard bone measurement. Once standard bone measurement[7] is missed, all the point locations will be missed; if the point locations are missed, then moxibustion and acupuncture will not only be ineffective but they will also certainly harm people. So the sages established standard bone measurements to teach later generations. It is not an easy method.

Books on the channels and network vessels, and methods of moxibustion and acupuncture have accumulated in numerous volumes, circulated widely in the world, and are well-known to all. Lots of them have benefited scholars. However, sometimes books do not conform to the meaning of the Classic.[8]

或曰：視此書，大凡（凡）的張介賓而議，汝曾有讎於張氏歟。抑按景岳者，明朝醫家之孤霍，德高，才智豐而天下顯名之人也。合靈素二經之類，照己之見識，著二經之注，間啟發蘊奧矣。其功績至大哉，舉世而賞焉。後學講二經者，多賴於類經也。汝今舉張氏之說以為非而議者，恐闊人之情而不可也。予應之曰：雖智者也不能無一失也。凡（凡）是為是，非為非者，天下之通論也。

Someone might say: When reading this book, in most cases, you targeted Zhāng Jièbīn[9] for criticism; do you hate Master Zhāng? Note that Zhāng Jīngyuè, was a doctor of the *Míng* dynasty who acted on his own. He was virtuous, intelligent, and world famous. He combined *Líng Shū* and *Sù Wèn* according to his own understanding, wrote annotations to these two classics, and also explained them profoundly. His achievement is so great and he was appreciated by the whole world. When later scholars talk about these two classics, they usu-

---

7. The term 骨度 *standard bone measurement* comes from *Nèi Jīng*. It refers to proportional measurement using anatomical landmarks, usually involving palpable features of the bones.

8. "The Classic" (*jīng* 經) in this book indicates *Huáng Dì Nèi Jīng* 《黃帝内經》 (The Yellow Emperor's Inner Classic), compiled during Spring and Autumn Period through the Warring States Period (1st century BCE).

9. Zhāng Jièbīn 張介賓 (1563–1640) was also named Zhāng Jīngyuè 張景岳. He was a famous doctor of the *Míng* dynasty.

ally rely on *Lèi Jīng*.[10] You give examples of Master Zhāng's theories which you think are wrong and discuss them. We are afraid that this will violate people's feelings and is not appropriate.

I respond: Even the wise are not always free from mistakes. True is true and false is false; this is the general rule of the world.

蓋按類經附翼，心主三焦命門，辨其下者，是之；高者，非之。又圖翼謂背俞篇，俠脊寸；形志篇，草度之法象，胸腹骨度之折法，肩至肘骨度之註，俱皆非經旨也。雖然舉世以為博識敏達，故不正其非而是之，信之者眾矣。

According to *Lèi Jīng Fù Yì*,[11] the pericardium, triple burner, and life gate are correctly identified as lower, and it is wrong to [identify them as] higher.[12] And all [the items below] mentioned in *Lèi Jīng Tú Yì*[13] are not the meaning of the Classic: the paravertebral measurement of *Bèi Shù Piān*,[14] the image of straw

---

10. *Lèi Jīng* 《 類經 》 (The Classified Classic) was written by Zhāng Jiebīn (1624, *Míng*).
11. *Lèi Jīng Fù Yì* 《 類經附翼 》 (Appendix for the Classified Classic) was written by Zhāng Jiebīn (1624, *Míng*). This sentence is probably commenting on the chapter called *Sān Jiāo Bāo Luò Mìng Mén Biàn* (Identification on Triple burner, Pericardium and Life Gate) in Volume 3.
12. In Volume 3 of *Lèi Jīng Fù Yì*, in the chapter called *Sān Jiāo Bāo Luò Mìng Mén Biàn* (Identification on Triple burner, Pericardium and Life Gate), Zhāng Jiebīn said that life gate may refer to the anterior yīn (the genitals) instead of the right kidney as stated in *Nán Jīng*. Thus, that makes the location lower. The author of this book, Cùnshàng Zōngzhàn, does not agree with this, nor with many of the other things Zhāng Jiebīn wrote.
13. *Lèi Jīng Tú Yì* 《 類經圖翼 》 (Illustrated Appendix for the Classified Classic) was written by Zhāng Jiebīn in *Míng* dynasty (1624).
14. *Bèi Shù Piān* 背俞篇 indicates *Líng Shū· Bèi Shù Piān* 《 靈樞· 背俞篇 》 (Magic Pivot Chapter 51, The Back Transport Points).

measurement[15] in *Xíng Zhì Piān*,[16] his standard bone measurement method for the chest and abdomen, and his annotation on standard bone measurement from the shoulder to the elbow. Even so, the whole world thought Zhāng Jīngyuè was knowledgeable and intelligent; they do not want to correct him but praise him instead. A lot of people trust him.

余曾嘆其以謬傳誤，故為吾子第著此書，名曰骨度正誤圖
說。不敢有仇於張氏，不得已也。篇未草度之法象，別以國
字和解，而便於初學童蒙云爾。

I have sighed that Zhāng Jīngyuè passed on these errors, so I wrote this book which is named *Gǔ Dù Zhèng Wù Tú Shuō* (Correcting Errors in Standard Bone Measurement with Illustrations) for my apprentices. I dare not despise Master Zhāng, but I have no choice. At the end of this book, there is diagram of straw (string) measurement with additional explanations in the national language [Japanese]. It is easy and convenient for beginners.

延享元年甲子十一月冬至日
村上親方宗占自敘

On the winter solstice day in the eleventh lunar month of the *jiǎ zǐ* year, the first year of Yánxiǎng's reign (1744), written by Cūnshàng Qīnfāng Zōngzhàn[17] himself

---

15. Straw measurement: An ancient way of locating certain points involved taking a long piece of straw or grass, measuring one part of the body, and using that measurement on another body part. The measured length is often folded to find a specific proportion of that length. This was used in *Sù Wèn· Xuè Qì Xíng Zhì Piān* and will be discussed in more detail below. Modern people are more likely to use string than straw. This method seems to be more popular in Japan today than in other places.
16. *Xíng Zhì Piān* 形志篇 indicates *Sù Wèn· Xuè Qì Xíng Zhì Piān* 《素問· 血 氣形志篇》 (Plain Questions Chapter 24, Qì and Blood (of the Channels) and Body and Mind).
17. Cūnshàng Qīnfāng Zōngzhàn 村上親方宗占 (Jp: Murakami, Sōsen Chika Masa) is Cūnshàng Zōngzhàn 村上宗占 (Jp: Murakami, Sōsen).

骨度正誤跋

Epilogue[18] for Correcting Errors in
Standard Bone Measurement

醫，民命所系，任重業博。為其術，內經為本，方藥為末，病論定而治療立，本末明而治療施。譬諸大匠作於廣廈堂宇，規矩準繩，得心應手，無施而不可也。故醫，國濟天下之名也。

Doctors who are responsible for people's life shoulder a heavy responsibility and must be knowledgeable in their field. To learn their skills, *Nèi Jīng* is the root while formulas and herbs are the branch. After the discussion of diseases is settled, treatment will be determined. When root and branch are understood, treatment can be carried out. Just like a master carpenter building a huge mansion, proficient with the compass and the square, there is nothing he cannot build. Like this, doctors are famous for their dedication to the country.

漢唐之間，諸名家出而從內經，有不失其義者矣。歷世到今日，醫家者流，勃然於世，立功爭名。診候之務，摩頂放踵無不盡，惟方是求，惟治是求。蓋治療之要，雖在於方藥，捨本務末，雖多奚為乎。

During the *Hàn* and *Táng* dynasties, all the famous scholars that came forth followed *Nèi Jīng*, and there were scholars who did not miss its meaning. From past generations until now, doctors have spread their schools of thought vigorously in the world, rendering service and striving for fame. Devoting themselves to examination and diagnosis, endlessly serving others and sacrificing themselves, only seeking formulas and only seeking treatment [not seeking the root]. Even though the essence of the treatment relies on the formulas and herbs, even if someone who abandons the root and strives for the branch does more, he will have no accomplishments.

---

18. While an epilogue is usually placed at the end of a book, this section is called an epilogue but is found here in the text.

同寮宗占，平素讀內經，精力過絕人，遂得其旨統，嘗著骨
度正誤。又素問血氣形志篇，草度之文，簡約而旨意深淵，
讀者難焉；類經草度解，雖張氏聰慧辨博，未盡焉；於是
乎，草度之方象出圖而書於所，得以辨解之，大發明經旨，
無餘蘊矣，使學者易曉指掌，璨目也，發先輩之所未發也，
誠不朽之確言也。

When my colleague Zōngzhàn read *Nèi Jīng*, his energy surpassed others, so he grasped its meaning and wrote *Gǔ Dù Zhèng Wù*. The section on straw (string) measurement in *Sù Wèn· Xue Qi Xíng Zhì Pian* is simple but profound, and readers have found it difficult. As for the explanation of straw (string) measurement in *Lèi Jīng*, even though Master Zhāng Jièbīn was intelligent and knowledgeable, he was unable to [explain it] thoroughly. Thus, the diagram of straw (string) measurement given here is able to explain it. This book greatly expounds the decree of the Classic without holding anything back and lets the scholar easily understand it. It brightens the eyes and expounds the [information] in a way that previous generations have not been able. These are really immortal words.

嗚呼！經之蘊奧，非闇記研究日久，豈可其得乎。骨度正
誤，形志篇，草度方解，合而著之，發張氏之未備，而遂成
一家言者也。

Alas! Regarding the stored-up mysteries of the Classic, how can [anyone] understand them without doing lengthy research and memorization? *Gǔ Dù Zhèng Wù* combines *Xíng Zhì Piān* with annotations on straw (string) measurement. It explains what Master Zhāng was unable to complete, and has become a [new] school of thought.

寶歷二年壬申五月七日與忠廣玄伸書於東都茅坡園

The seventh day of the fifth lunar month of the *rén shēn* year, the second year of Bǎolì's reign (1752), written by Yǔzhōng Guǎngxuán[19] in Máopō Garden in Dōngdū

---

19. Yǔzhōng Guǎngxuán 與忠廣玄伸 Yochū, Kōgenshin: No information is currently available about this person.

凡例
Notes on Usage

一先輩數多出銅人形圖畫矣。予嘗視其圖畫，間有差謬，故
初學迷其正疑。予以所學於師，為子弟出圖畫焉。於胸腹手
足，附刻骨度之尺寸，而使俞穴知分寸也。負附刻而知骨度
穴處之尺寸，是發前人未發也。

Previous generations mostly followed the diagrams of *Tóng Rén*.[20] I have seen
these diagrams and they have some mistakes, so the beginner may be confused as to whether they are correct or questionable. I have used what I have
learned from my master to draw diagrams for my apprentices. I have attached
engravings of the *chǐ* and *cùn* standard measurements for the bones of the
chest, abdomen, and limbs, so that the measurement for finding points will be
clear. See the attached engravings to know the measurement for points located
within the bone measurements. This expands what previous generations have
left unexplained.

一 篇中獨的張景岳而議焉，不敢有讎焉。按，晉自皇莆謐
下至明世，豪杰起而經絡之書今不乏，蓋各有得失，今不暇
儀焉。其中景岳尤為博識顯名之人，舉世賞焉，然錯骨度，
故俞穴之分寸亦間差，有不似景岳之聰明也。未聞有正其非
者，卻而是之者有焉。予曾嘆傳誤於世，斯以為敵，而為議
焉。

In the book, I alone target Zhāng Jǐngyuè for criticism but I dare not despise
him. Note that from Huángfǔ Mì of the *Jìn* dynasty down to the *Míng* dynasty,
heroes have arisen and there were plenty of books on the channels and network vessels. Each had its pros and cons, but the meaning cannot be seen today.

---

20. This refers to *Tóng Rén Shù Xuè Zhēn Jiǔ Tú Jīng* 《銅人腧穴針灸圖
經》(The Bronze Statues Illustrated Classic of Acupuncture Points) by Wáng
Wéiyī 王維一 (1027, *Sòng*).

Among them, Zhāng Jǐngyuè was the most knowledgeable and well-known person, and was admired by the whole world. However, he misunderstood standard bone measurement, so his measurement for the points was somewhat wrong; it does not seem like Zhāng Jǐngyuè was so intelligent. I never heard that anyone corrected his mistakes, but there are those who praise him. I sigh that he passed on the wrong information to the world, so I discuss him as if he were an opponent.

一 銅人形圖系彩，以其藏府之色，由於素問經絡論也，藏經濃府經薄。今所彩，肺經銀○大腸經胡粉○心經朱○小腸經丹○心胞經紫○三焦經薄紫○腎經黑○膀胱經薄黑○脾經黃○胃經薄黃○肝經青○膽經綠青○督脈金○任脈銀，視其系彩，而可知藏府之經行矣 。

The diagrams from *Tóng Rén* are in color;[21] the colors of the organs came from *Sù Wèn·Jīng Luò Lùn*.[22] The colors of the *zàng*-organs are darker, and the colors of the *fǔ*-organs are lighter. The colors used here are: lung channel - silver; large intestine channel – lead white;[23] heart channel - dark red; small intestine channel - red; pericardium channel - purple; sānjiāo channel - light purple; kidney channel - black; urinary bladder channel - light black; spleen channel - yellow; stomach channel - light yellow; liver channel - green; gall bladder channel - green blue; dū vessel - gold; rèn vessel - silver. When looking at the color, one can know to which organ the channel pathway belongs.

凡例終

End of Notes on Usage

21. The original *Tóng Rén* did not have color illustrations, although perhaps the author had a later edition that was colored in. At the time this was written, it is likely that it was hand colored (not printed with color). He probably instructed his students to color the organs and channels as listed here.
22. This refers to *Sù Wèn* 《 素問 》 (Plain Questions), Chapter 57.
23. *Hú fěn* (lead subcarbonate) is a mineral, also named *lead white*.

銅人形總圖

General Diagrams from the Tóng Rén Figure

俞穴中

Among acupuncture points:

三角者禁針	四角者禁灸
Points marked with △ are contraindicated for needling.	Points marked with □ are contraindicated for moxibustion.

Ill.1

玉堂
靈墟 膺窗 胸鄉
膻中 天池 天溪 青靈 天泉 尺澤
神封 乳中
彧中 步郎 乳根 少海 曲澤
鳩尾 不容 期門
巨闕 幽門 日月
上脘 通谷 承滿
中脘 陰都 梁門
建里 石關 關門 腹哀
下脘 商曲 太乙 章門
水分 肓俞 滑肉門
神闕 中注 天樞 大橫 帶脈
陰交 四滿 外陵 腹結 胝骨
氣海 水道 大巨 五樞
石門 五樞 維道
關元 氣穴 府舍
中極 大赫 衝門
曲骨 極 歸來 居髎
橫骨 衝會
陰廉
急脈
五里

Ill.2

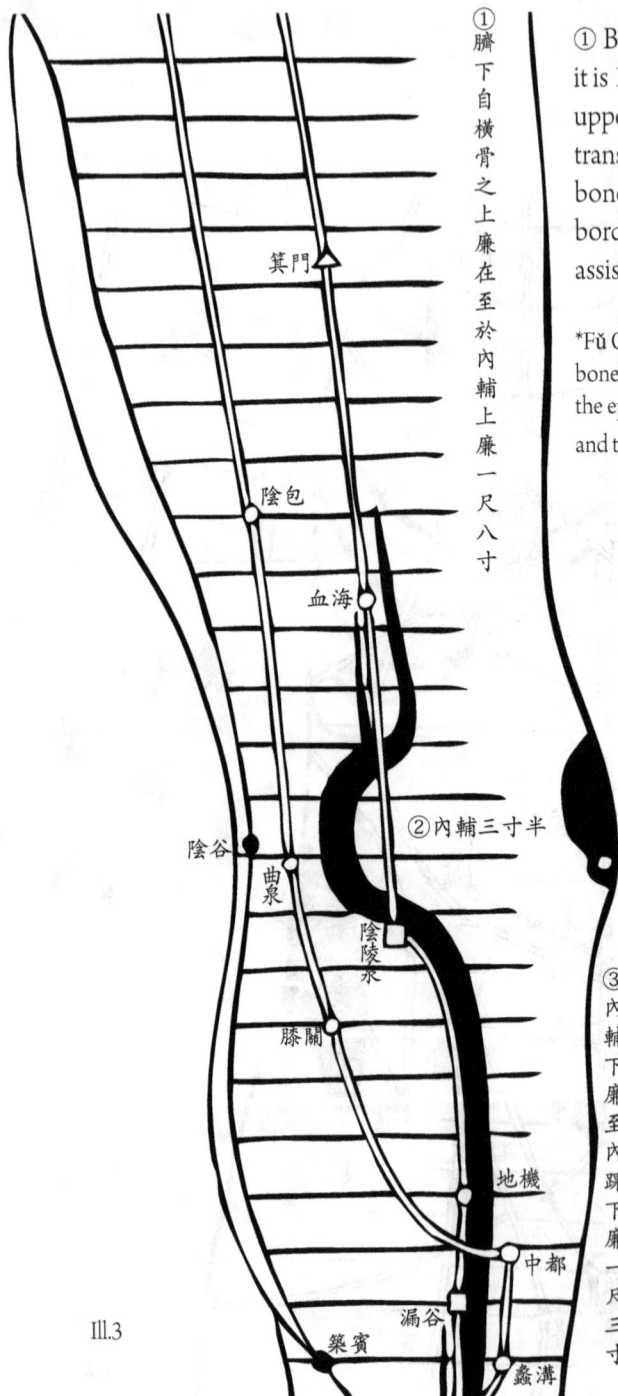

① 臍下自橫骨之上廉在至於內輔上廉一尺八寸

箕門

陰包

血海

②內輔三寸半

陰谷

曲泉

陰陵泉

膝關

地機

中都

漏谷

築賓

蠡溝

③內輔下廉至內踝下廉一尺三寸

① Below the umbilicus, it is 1.8 chǐ from the upper border of the transverse bone (pubic bone) to the upper border of the medial assisting bone.*

*Fǔ Gǔ 輔骨 (assisting bone), the region formed by the epicondyle of the femur and the condyle of the tibia.

② [The height of the] medial assisting bone is 3.5 cùn.

③ It is 1.3 chǐ from the lower border of the medial assisting bone to the lower border of the medial malleolus.

Ill.3

① It is 1.2 chǐ from Qū Zé 曲澤 (PC 3)to Dà Líng 大陵 (PC 7).

② It is 8 cùn from Dà Líng 大陵 (PC 7) to the tip of the middle finger (see other oral instructions).

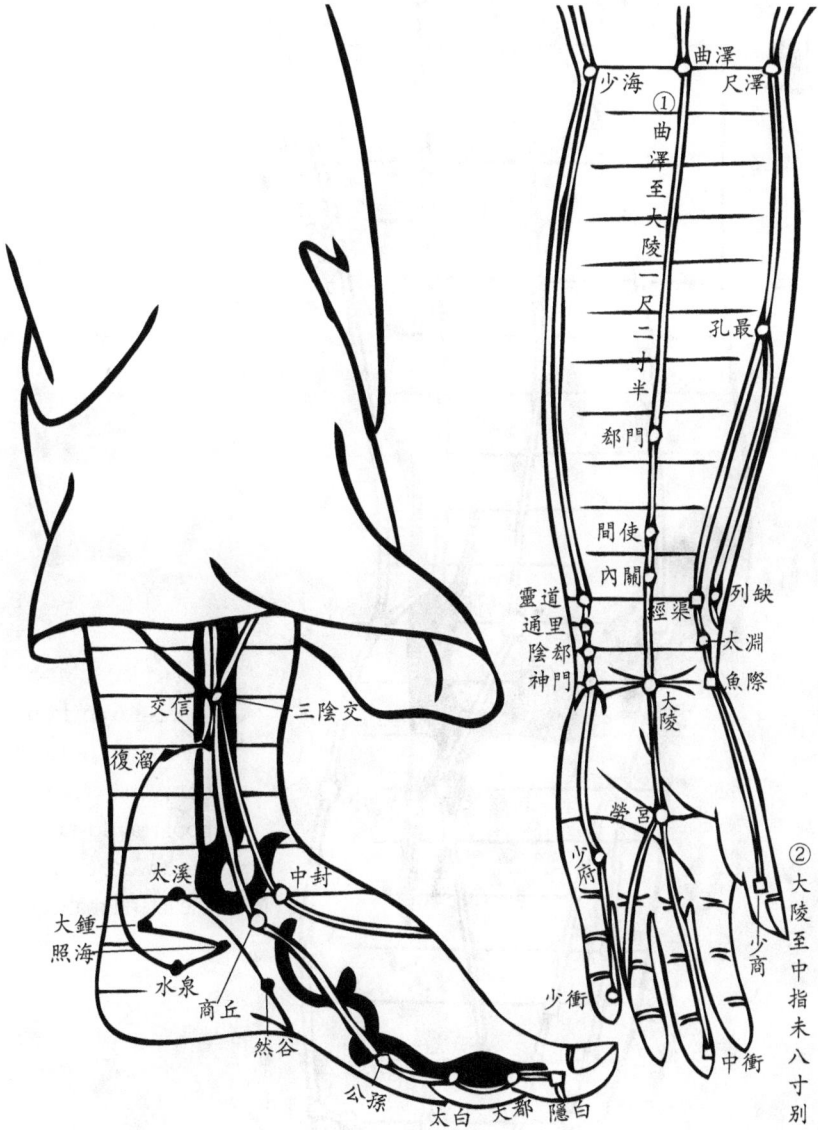

Ill.4

23

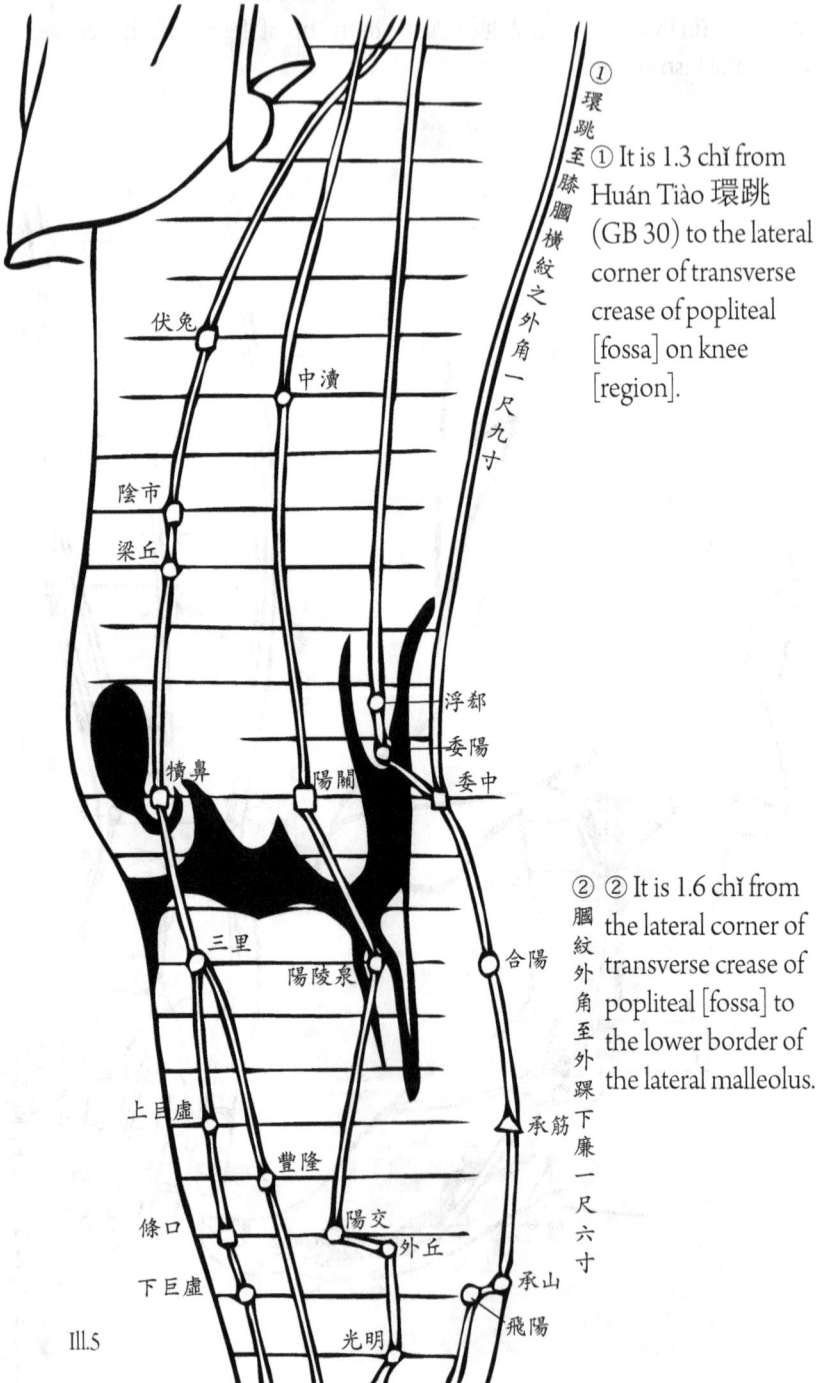

① 環跳至膝膕橫紋之外角一尺九寸

① It is 1.3 chǐ from Huán Tiào 環跳 (GB 30) to the lateral corner of transverse crease of popliteal [fossa] on knee [region].

伏兔

中瀆

陰市

梁丘

浮郄

委陽

委中

犢鼻

陽關

② 膕紋外角至外踝下廉一尺六寸

② It is 1.6 chǐ from the lateral corner of transverse crease of popliteal [fossa] to the lower border of the lateral malleolus.

三里

陽陵泉

合陽

上巨虛

承筋

豐隆

條口

陽交

外丘

承山

下巨虛

飛陽

光明

Ill.5

小海
曲池

三里
上廉
下廉
四瀆
溫溜
支正
三陽絡
會宗　支溝
偏歷
外關
養老
陽谷　陽溪
陽池
腕骨
合谷
後溪
三間
中渚
前谷　液門
二間
商陽
少澤
行間
關衝
大敦
屬兌

陽輔
附陽
懸鍾
解溪
崑崙
僕參
丘墟
商陽
中脈
臨泣
金門
太衝
京骨
陰谷
俠溪
通谷
竅陰

Ill.6

25

Ill.7

① It is 1.3 chǐ from the axilla to the rib-sides.
② It is 6 cùn from the rib-sides to Huán Tiào 環跳 (GB 30).

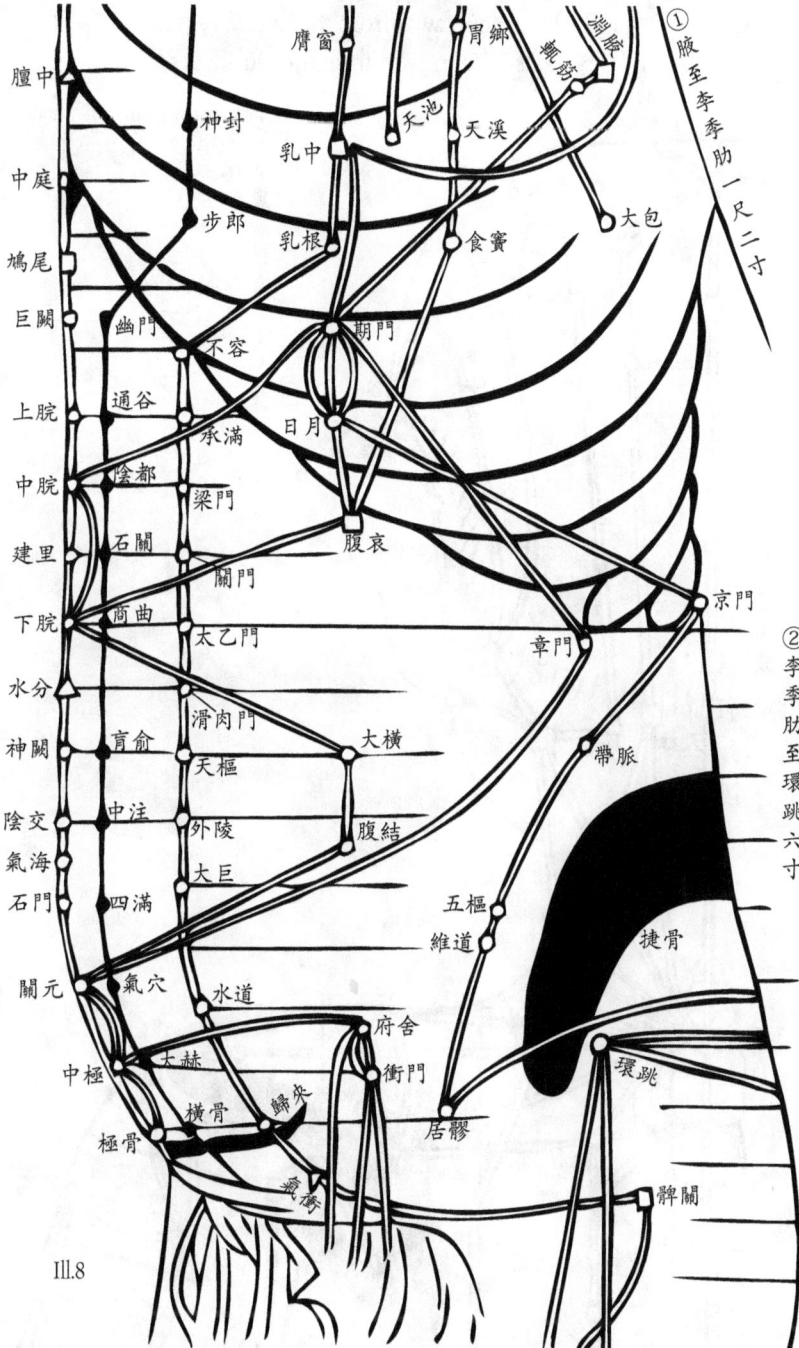

Ill.8

① Chéng Líng 承靈 (GB 18) is 2.1 cùn away from the Dū 督 vessel.

② Fēng Chí 風池 (GB 20) is 2 cùn away from the Dū 督 vessel.

③ Luò Què 絡卻 (UB 8) is 2.1 cùn away from the Dū 督 vessel.

④ Tiān Zhù 天柱 (UB 10) is 2.1 cùn away from the Dū 督 vessel.

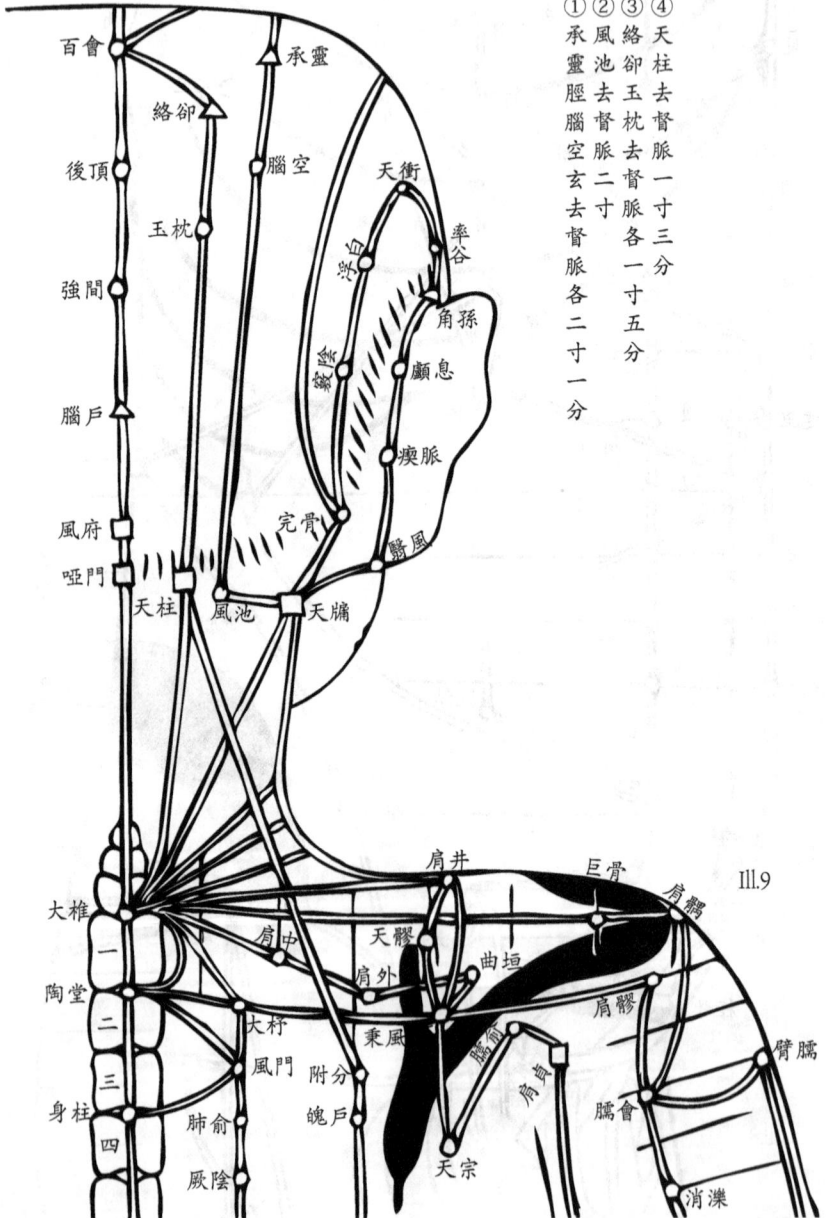

Ill.9

五 六 七 八 九 十 十一 十二 十三 十四 十五 十六 十七 十八 十九 二十

神道 靈臺 至陽 筋縮 脊中 懸樞 命門 陽關 腰俞 長強

心俞 膈俞 肝俞 膽俞 脾俞 胃俞 三焦俞 腎俞 大腸俞 上髎 次髎 中髎 下髎 小腸俞 膀胱俞 中膂內俞 白環俞 會陽

膏肓俞 神堂 譩譆 膈關 魂門 陽綱 意舍 胃倉 肓門 志室 胞肓 秩邊

環跳

五里 清冷淵 天井 肘髎 曲池 小海 三里

曲池至腕之陽谿一尺二寸半

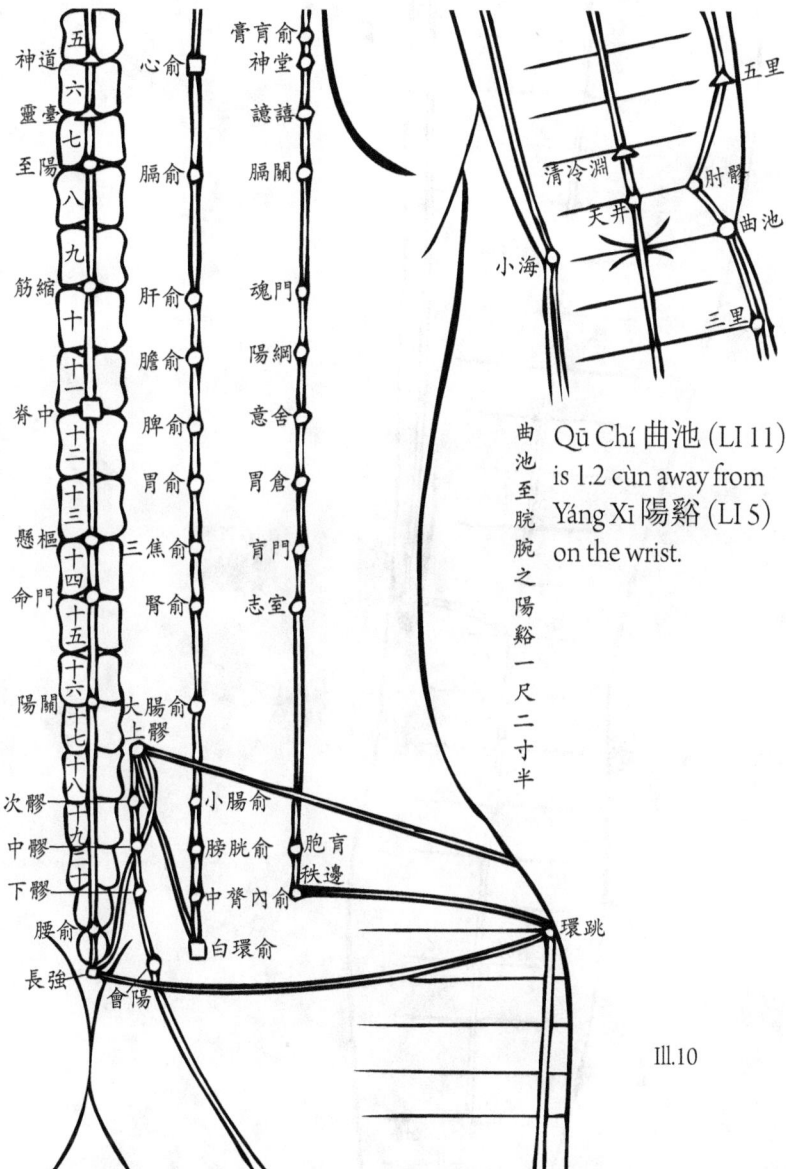

Qū Chí 曲池 (LI 11) is 1.2 cùn away from Yáng Xī 陽谿 (LI 5) on the wrist.

Ill.10

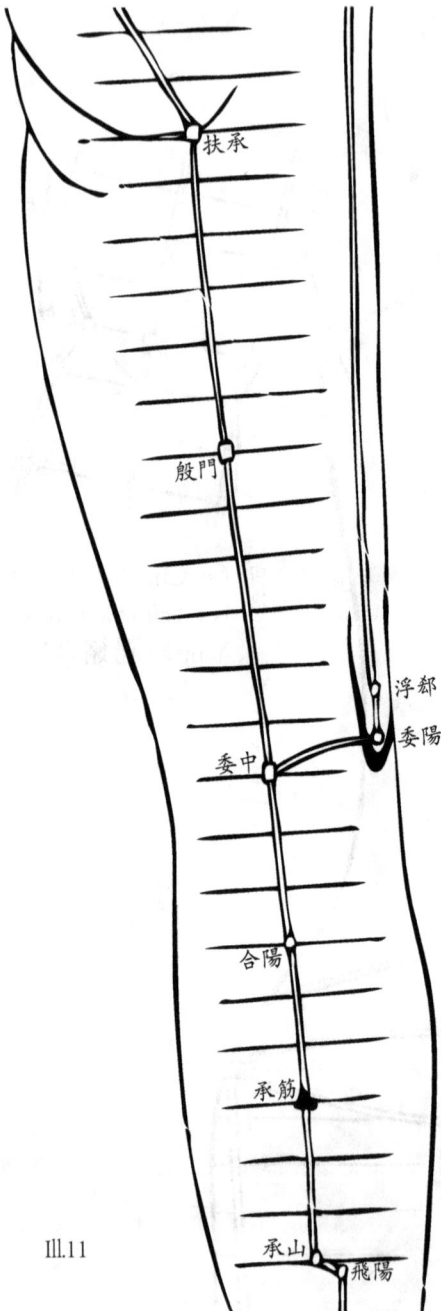

扶承

殷門

浮郄

委陽

委中

合陽

承筋

承山　飛陽

Ill.11

禁灸之穴歌（數唱而可記臆焉）
Song of Points Contraindicated for Moxibustion
(one can memorize this by singing it repeatedly)

禁灸之穴四十五，承光啞門及風府。
天柱素窌臨泣上，睛明攢竹迎香數。
禾窌顴窌紫竹空，頭維下關與脊中。
肩貞心俞白環俞，天牖人迎俱乳中。
周榮淵液并鳩尾，腹哀少商魚際位。
經渠天府及中衝，陽關陽池地五會。
隱白漏谷陰陵泉，條口犢鼻與陰市。
伏兔髀關委中穴，殷門申脈承扶忌。

There are forty-five points contraindicated for moxibustion:
Chéng Guāng (UB 6), Yǎ Mén (Dū 15), and Fēng Fǔ (Dū 16).
Tiān Zhù (UB 10), Sù Liáo (Dū 25), and Lín Qì (GB 15) are above;
Jīng Míng (UB 1), Zǎn Zhú (UB 2), and Yíng Xiāng (LI 20) will be counted.
Hé Líao (LI 19), Quán Líao (SI 18), and Zǐ Zhú Kōng (SJ 23);
Tóu Wéi (ST 8), Xià Guān (ST 7), and Jǐ Zhōng (Dū 6).
Jiān Zhēn (SI 9), Xīn Shù (UB 15), and Bái Huán Shù (UB 30);
Tiān Yǒu (SJ 16) and Rén Yíng (ST 9) combine with Rǔ Zhōng (ST 17).
Zhōu Róng (SP 20) and Yuān Yè (GB 22) with Jiū Wěi (Rèn 15);
Fù Āi (SP 16), and Shào Shāng (LU 11) is located with Yú Jì (LU 10).
Jīng Qú (LU 8), Tiān Fǔ (LU 3), and Zhōng Chōng (PC 9);
Yáng Guān (GB 33), Yáng Chí (SJ 4), and Dì Wǔ Huì (GB 42).
Yǐn Bái (SP 1), Lòu Gǔ (SP 7), and Yīn Líng Quán (SP 9);
Tiáo Kǒu (ST 38), Dú Bí (ST 35), and Yīn Shì (ST 33).
Fú Tù (ST 32), Bì Guān (ST 31), and Wěi Zhōng (UB 40);
Yīn Mén (UB 37) and Shēn Mài (UB 62) with Chéng Fǔ (UB 36)
are all contraindicated.

禁鍼之穴歌
Song of Points Contraindicated for Acupuncture

二十二穴不可鍼，
腦戶顖會及神庭，絡卻玉枕角孫穴，
顱顖承泣與承靈，神道靈臺膻中忌，
水分神闕并會陰，橫骨氣衝手五里，
箕門承筋及青靈，更加臂上三陽絡 。

Twenty-two points cannot be needled:
Nǎo Hù (Dū 17), Xìn Huì (Dū 22), and Shéng Tíng (Dū 24).
Luò Què (UB 8) and Yù Zhěn (UB 9) with Jiǎo Sūn (SJ 20);
Lú Xìn (SJ 19), Chéng Qì (ST 1), and Chéng Líng (GB 18).
Shén Dào (Dū 11), Líng Tái (Dū 10), and Dàn Zhōng (Rèn 17)
are contraindicated.
So are Shuǐ Fēn (Rèn 9), Shén Què (Rèn 8), and Huì Yīn (Rèn 1);
Héng Gǔ (KI 11), Qì Chōng (ST 30), and Shǒu Wǔ Lǐ (LI 13);
Jī Mén (SP 11) and Chéng Jīng (UB 56) with Qīng Líng (HT 2);
Plus Sān Yáng Luò (SJ 8) on the arms.

婦人常禁石門穴，合谷三陰交孕忌 。
若深肩井人悶倒，補三里穴必平安 。
莫深刺云門鳩尾，缺盆并客主人穴 。

Shí Mén (Rèn 5) is contraindicated in women;
Hé Gǔ (LI 4) and Sān Yīn Jiāo (SP 6) are avoided in pregnancy.
Needling Jiān Jǐng (GB 21) deeply induces unconsciousness;
Supplementing Sān Lǐ (ST 36) will keep one healthy.
Do not prick Yún Mén (LU 2) or Jiū Wěi (Rèn 15) too deeply;
Along with Quē Pén (ST 12) and Kè Zhǔ Rén (GB 3).

附刻於胸腹者，骨度也，數之可知骨度矣 。

The attached diagrams mark the standard bone measurement on the chest and abdomen. By counting it, one can learn the standard bone measurements.

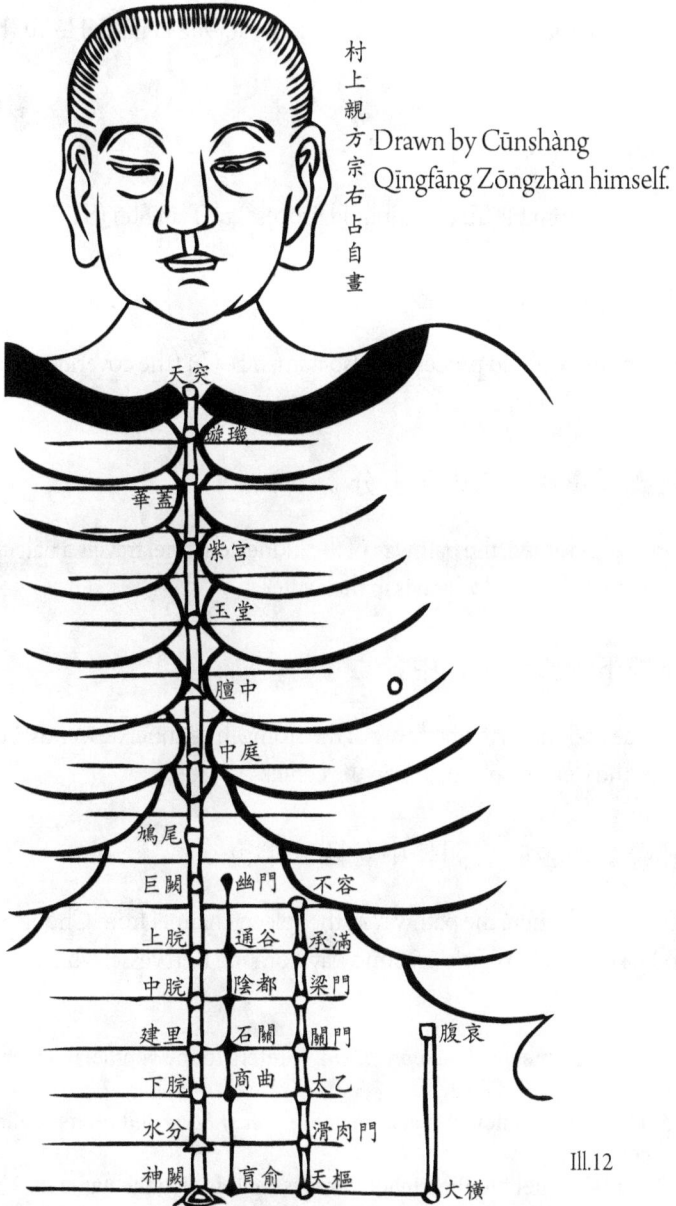

村上親方宗右占自畫

Drawn by Cūnshàng Qīngfāng Zōngzhàn himself.

Ill.12

正誤，此內經之本旨也矣：
Correcting Errors: this is the original meaning of *Nèi Jīng*:

自缺盆中天突至髑骭九寸。

It is 9 cùn from Tiān Tū (Rèn 22) which is at Quē Pén[24] to Hé Yú (the xiphoid process).[25]

自髑骭至天樞八寸。

It is 8 cùn from Hé Yú (the xiphoid process) to Tiān Shū (ST 25).

髑骭一名蔽骨，一名鳩尾。

Hé Yú (the xiphoid process) is also named Bì Gǔ (the covering bone); another name is Jīu Wěi.[26]

腎經循腹者去任中各五分。

On the abdomen, the pathway of the kidney channel travels a half cùn away from the Rèn vessel which is in the center.

胃經下行腹者去任中各二寸。

On the abdomen, the pathway of the stomach channel descends 2 cùn away from the Rèn vessel which is in the center.

脾經衝門至腹哀開任中各四寸半也。

On the abdomen, the pathway of the spleen channel from Chōng Mén (SP 12) to Fù Āi (SP 16) travels 4.5 cùn away from the Rèn vessel which is in the center.

---

24. Quē Pén means the *empty basin*. It refers to the supraclavicular fossa and is also the name of ST 12.
25. Hé Yú is an ancient name meaning *breast bone* and refers to the xiphoid process.
26. Jīu Wěi refers to the xiphoid process and is also the name of Rèn 15.

胸腹背橫寸方者皆用兩乳八寸 。

All transverse cùn measurements on the chest and abdomen use [the distance between] the nipples as 8 cùn.

此內經之本旨也。
This is the original meaning of *Nèi Jīng*.

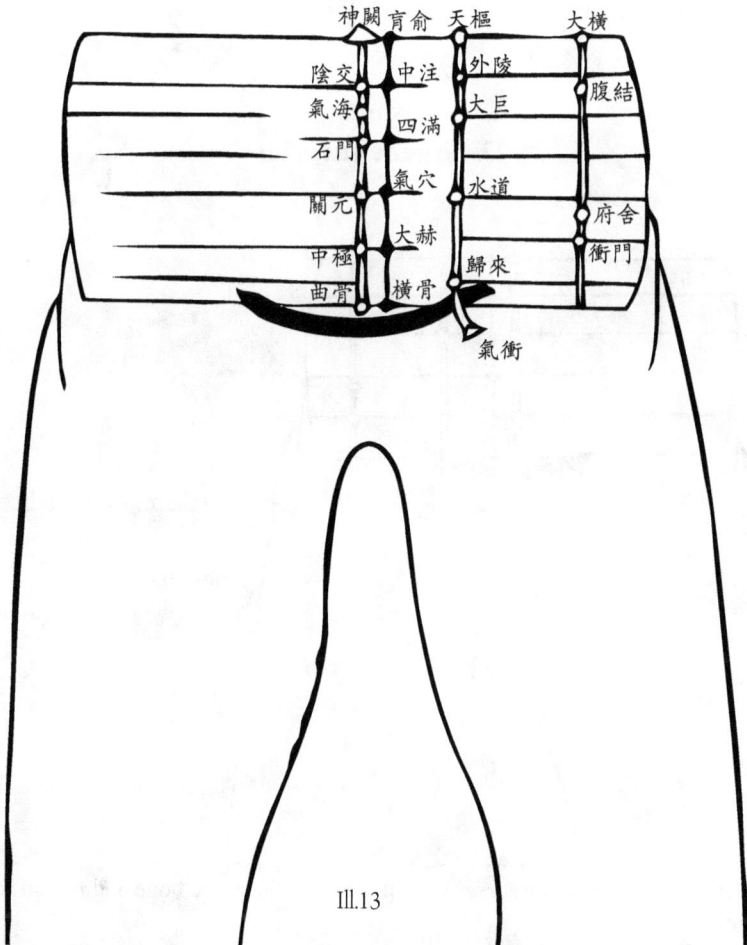

神闕 肓俞 天樞　　大橫

陰交　中注　外陵

氣海　四滿　大巨　　腹結

石門

關元　氣穴　水道

　　　大赫　　　　府舍

中極　　　歸來　　衝門

曲骨　橫骨

氣衝

Ill.13

自天樞至橫骨六寸半，蓋腎經與任脈可為臍下於五寸也，脾胃之兩經者可取於六寸半矣。

It is 6.5 cùn from Tiān Shū (ST 25) to Héng Gǔ.[27] The pathways of the kidney channel and the Rèn vessel below the umbilicus are 5 cùn long. The pathways of the spleen and stomach channels below the umbilicus are 6.5 cùn long.

如此臍下之骨度諸經皆為五寸，則脾胃之兩經穴處不居本位也，故為誤焉。

If the standard bone measurement for all channels below the umbilicus is now considered to be 5 cùn, then the points of spleen and stomach channels are not found in their original location. Therefore this is wrong.

異說
Divergent Theories

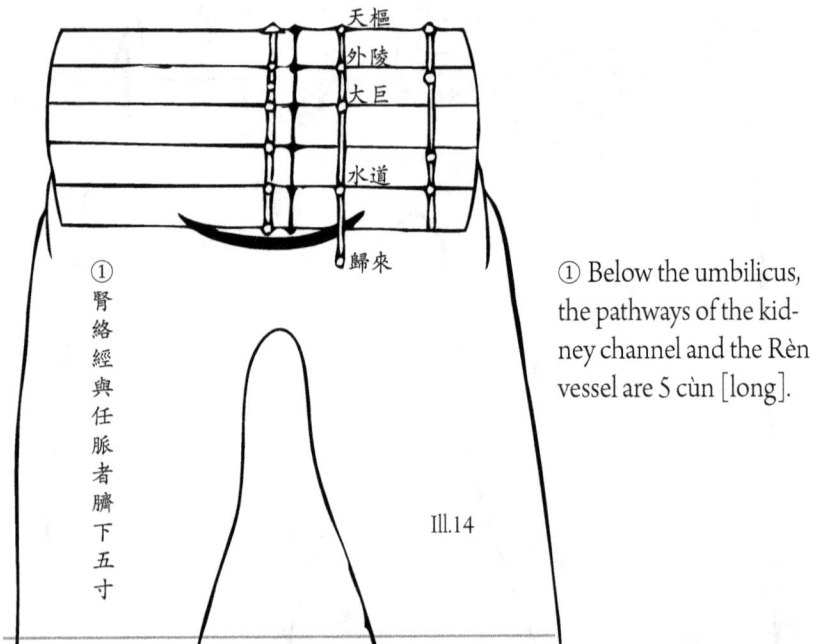

① Below the umbilicus, the pathways of the kidney channel and the Rèn vessel are 5 cùn [long].

Ill.14

27. Héng Gǔ means *transverse bone*. It refers to the pubic bone and is also the name of KI 11.

近世所謂歸來當橫骨下者誤也。按：歸來在橫骨之上廉也，
氣衝者在歸來之下，橫骨之下廉也。歸來在橫骨下，則氣衝
無可著地矣。圖翼誤骨度也。

Recently, the point called Guī Lái (ST 29) has been located below Héng Gǔ
(the transverse bone); this is wrong.

Comments: Guī Lái (ST 29) is on the upper border of Héng Gǔ; Qì Chōng
(ST 30) is below Guī Lái (ST 29), and is on the lower border of Héng Gǔ. If
Guī Lái (ST 29) is below Héng Gǔ, there is no place for Qì Chōng (ST 30). *Tú
Yì* made a mistake in standard bone measurement.

近世人臍下之骨度，諸經等量於五寸者，非也矣。

Recently, people [say that] the standard bone measurement below the umbilicus equals 5 cùn for all channels; this is wrong.

正說 （此內經之本旨也矣）
Correct Theories (This is the original meaning of *Nèi Jīng*)

骨度篇類經註曰：肩者肩端也云。是以今世之醫肩端自肩髃
至曲池為一尺七寸者，甚誤也。

An annotation on *Gǔ Dù Piān* in *Lèi Jīng* says: *Shoulder* means the end of the
shoulder. Because of this, doctors today are quite wrong when they say that
there are 1.7 chǐ from the end of the shoulder at Jiān Yú (LI 15) to Qū Chí (LI
11).

骨度篇曰：肩至肘一尺七寸者，脊中至肘後骨尖為一尺七寸
矣。自肘後骨尖至腕橫紋一尺二寸半，自腕橫紋至中指本節
四寸，自中指本節至末四寸。經曰：四寸半。按，半字衍
也，可削。蓋此章別有口傳矣。

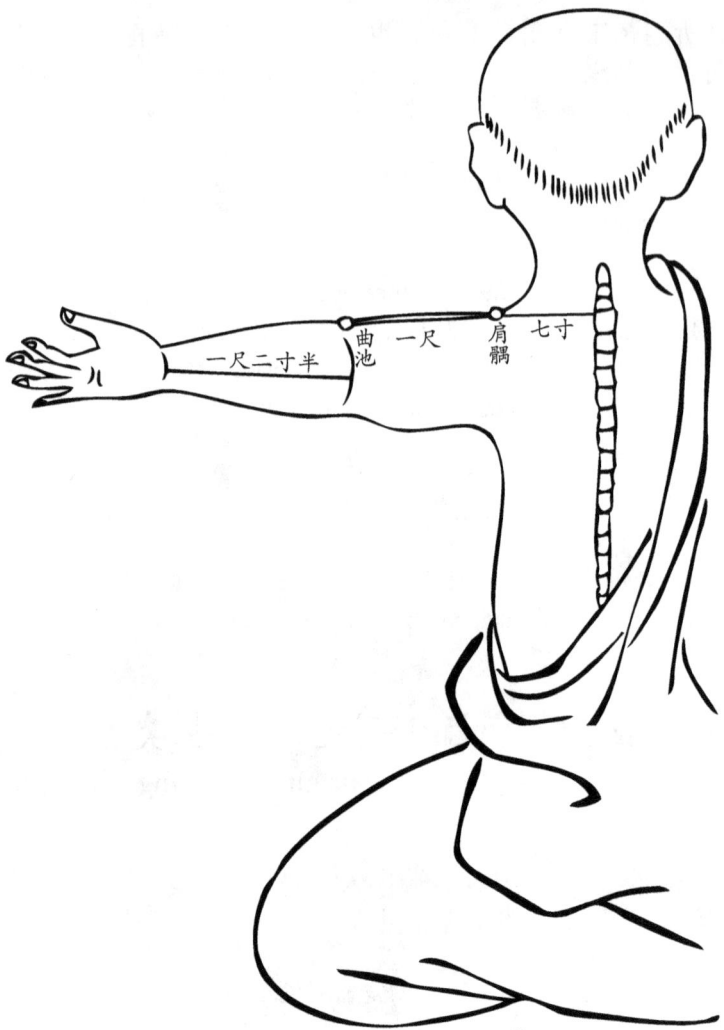

一尺二寸半　　曲池　一尺　肩髃　七寸

Ill.15

Gǔ Dù Piān says: It is 1.7 chǐ from the shoulder to the elbow. This means from the center of the spine to the tip of the bone at the posterior aspect of the elbow.[28]

---

28. The word shoulder (*jiān* 肩), as in English can refer to the shoulder joint or can include a much broader area. The author is addressing a dispute as to whether the word *shoulder* in *Gǔ Dù Piān* refers to the region of Jiān Yú (LI 15) at the end of the shoulder or something else. The author feels *shoulder* refers to the region of Dà Zhuī (Dū 14).

- From the tip of the bone at the posterior aspect of the elbow to the wrist crease is 1.25 chỉ.

- From the wrist crease to the base joint of the middle finger is 4 cùn.

- From the base joint of the middle finger to its tip is 4 cùn. The Classic says it is 4.5 cùn.

Comment: *Half* [*bàn* 半 or 0.5 cùn] is wrong and needs to be removed.[29]

This chapter has other oral instructions.[30]

29. The reason the author believes that the word *half* should be removed is discussed in a footnote in Chapter 8.
30. This book seems to have been written for the author's students and disciples. In a few places, it mentions oral instructions. This may have been to keep some of his teaching secret, or it may have been because some things are easier to show students than to write down in a book.

正說（此內經之本旨也矣。）

Correct Theory: This is the original meaning of the *Nèi Jīng*.

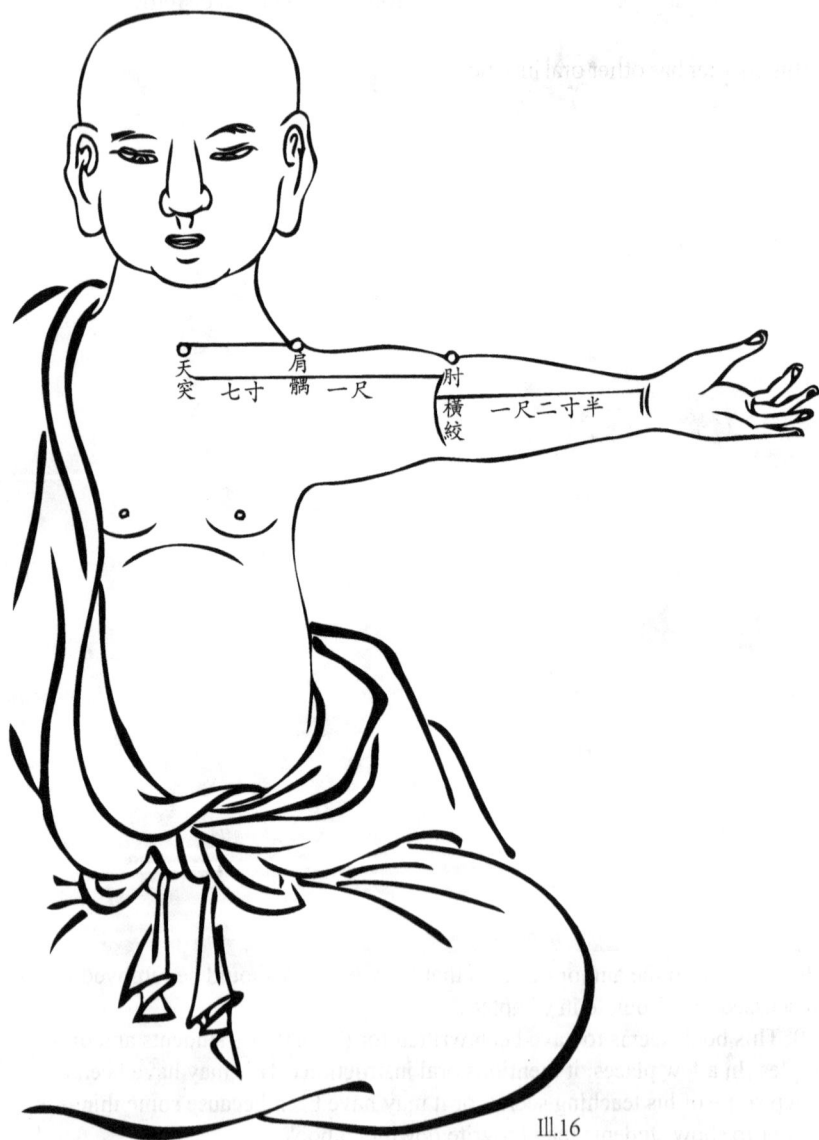

Ill.16

自腕之橫紋至中指之末八寸。

It is 8 cùn from the transverse crease of the wrist to the tip of the middle finger.

自肘紋至腕之橫紋一尺二寸半。

It is 1.25 chǐ from the elbow crease to the transverse crease of the wrist.

自天突至肘之橫紋長一尺七寸。

It is 1.7 chǐ from Tiān Tū (Rèn 22) to the transverse crease of the elbow.

十四經發揮表圖
Diagram from *Elaboration on the Fourteen Channels*

肝經繞乎陰器圖
Diagram of the liver channel encircling the yīn organ [genitals]

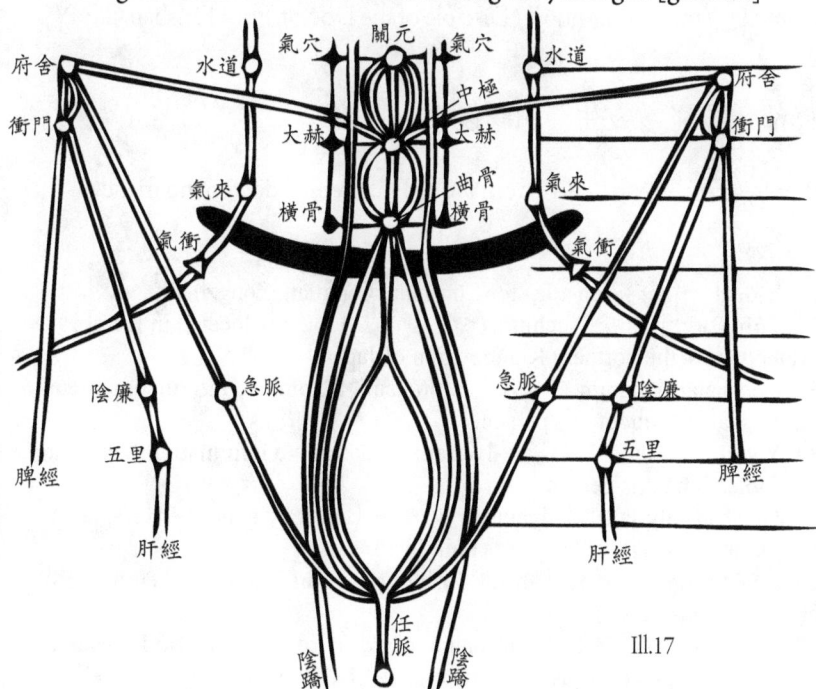

氣穴　關元　氣穴　水道
府舍　水道　　　　　　中極　　府舍
衝門　　　　　　太赫　太赫　　　衝門
大赫　　　　　　曲骨　氣來
氣來　　　　横骨　横骨
氣衝　　　　　　　　　　氣衝

陰廉　急脈　　　急脈　陰廉
脾經　五里　　　　　　五里　脾經
肝經　　　　　　　　　肝經

陰蹻　任脈　陰蹻

Ill.17

骨度正誤圖說

Correcting Errors in Standard Bone Measurement
with Illustrations (*Gǔ Dù Zhèng Wù Tú Shuō*)

土甫城醫員　一得子村上親方宗占　　　著

Written by Cūnshàng Qīngfāng Zōngzhàn, also called Yīdézǐ[31] - Doctor from Túfǔ City[32]

男　　村上宗珉

Mister Cūnshàng Zōngmín[33]

飯山城醫員　門人　巖崎隆碩　　輯

Edited by Yánqí Nóngshuò[34] - Disciple of the Doctor, from Fànshān City[35]

東都　隱醫　友生　加藤俊夫　　校

Proofread by Jiāténg Jùnfū[36] from Dōng Dū,[37] retired doctor and friend

---

31. Yīdézǐ 一得子 is an alias for Cūnshàng Qīngfāng Zōngzhàn.
32. Túfǔ City 土浦城 Tsuchiura (つちうらし) is a city located in Ibaraki Prefecture, in the northern Kantō region of Japan.
33. Cūnshàng Zōngmín 村上宗珉 Murakami, Sōmin: No information is currently available about this person.
34. Yánqí Nóngshuò 巖崎隆碩 Iwasaki, Ryūseki: No information is currently available about this person.
35. Fànshān City 飯山城 Iiyama (いいやまし), a city in northern Nagano Prefecture now. The old city was built in 1564.
36. Jiāténg Jùnfū 加藤俊夫 Katō, Toshio: No information is currently available about this person.
37. Dōng Dū 東都 Tō To (a nickname for Edo): Edo (えど), also Romanized as Jedo, Yedo or Yeddo, is the former name of Tokyo.

二

Chapter 2

骨度篇曰：缺盆至髑骭九寸，髑骭至天樞八寸，天樞至橫骨
六寸半云云。

Gǔ Dù Piān says: It is 9 cùn from Quē Pén (the supraclavicular fossa) to Hé Yú (the xiphoid process).[38] It is 8 cùn from Hé Yú (the xiphoid process) to Tiān Shū (ST 25). It is 6.5 cùn from Tiān Shū (ST 25) to Héng Gǔ (the transverse bone or pubic bone).[39]

類經圖翼胸腹折法曰：胸腹折法，直寸以中行為主。自缺盆
中天突起至歧骨際上中庭穴止，折八寸四分；自髑骭上歧骨
際下至臍中折作八寸；自臍心下至毛際曲骨穴折作五寸也；
胸腹直寸法並依之云。

The measurement method for the chest and abdomen in *Lèi Jīng Tú Yì*, says: "The measurement method for the chest and abdomen: the vertical measurement mainly follows the midline.

---

38. In this and the next chapter, pay special attention to the words Hé Yú (the xiphoid process), Bì Gǔ (covering bone – another name for the xiphoid process according to the author), and Qí Gǔ (bone junction – the junction of the ribs with the xiphoid process). The author feels that people have confused the terms for the xiphoid process with the bone junction, leading to improper measurement. In Chapter 4, the author makes clear his opinion is that the xiphoid process is 0.6 cùn long and that the measurement should be to the lower tip of the xiphoid process. Confusing the xiphoid process with the bone junction then makes an error of 0.6 cùn in proportional measurement for both the chest and upper abdomen.

39. These are all vertical references. Some of these landmarks are at the midline and others are lateral to the midline, but only the vertical distance is counted. In other words, the sentence could be paraphrased in modern English as saying "It is 9 cùn from the level of the supraclavicular fossa to the level of the xiphoid process. It is 8 cùn from the level of the xiphoid process to the level of the umbilicus. It is 6.5 cùn from the level of the umbilicus to the level of the pubic bone."

- It measures 8.4 cùn from Tiān Tū (Rèn 22) in the center of Quē Pén (the supraclavicular fossa) to Zhōng Tíng (Rèn 16) on the border of Qí Gǔ (the bone junction).
- It measures 8 cùn from the border of Qí Gǔ at Hé Yú (the xiphoid process) down to the center of umbilicus.
- It measures 5 cùn from the center of the umbilicus to Qū Gǔ (Rèn 2) in the hairy region.

The vertical measurements on the chest and abdomen region should follow this."

按：此說非也，由張氏發此語以後，世醫從之者眾矣。又醫學綱目立異說，甚非也，非自誤而使學者誤焉。介賓、樓英二子素明經史，博通諸家之言而註內經也，多所發明，故今有助於醫家不少矣，雖然其於骨度有註解之誤也。二子之聰明如何如此哉！

Comments: This theory is wrong, but because Master Zhāng Jièbīn commented on it, lots of the doctors nowadays follow it. *Yī Xué Gāng Mù*[40] also has divergent theories which are incorrect. They not only made mistakes for themselves; they also confused other scholars. Both scholars, Zhāng Jièbīng and Lóu Yīng, usually understood the history of the classics. They were proficient in different schools of theory and they annotated *Nèi Jīng*; they expounded a lot of information and benefited a lot of doctors today. Even so, they made mistakes in their annotations on standard bone measurement. These two scholars were quite intelligent, so why did they do this!

按：周身之輸穴分寸者，以骨度量之也。骨度俞穴一差，則灸刺不徒益而施害於人也必矣，不可不慎也。

Comments: Standard bone measurement is used all over the body to determine the distances for locating points. Once the standard bone measurement for a point is wrong, acupuncture and moxibustion will not benefit people, and will also certainly damage them. We must be cautious.

---

40. *Yī Xué Gāng Mù* 《醫學綱目》 (Compendium of Medicine) was written by Lóu Yīng 楼英 (1332-1401) in 1565, *Míng* dynasty.

張氏曰：自髑骬上歧骨際下至臍心，謂八寸也。由是觀之，則歧骨際上至天突為九寸分明也。自張氏發此語以來，今之醫多本之也。

Master Zhāng Jièbīn said: From the border of Qí Gǔ (the bone junction) at Hé Yú (the xiphoid process) down to the center of umbilicus, the measurement is 8 cùn. So from this point of view, it is clear that from the border of Qí Gǔ up to Tiān Tū (Rèn 22) would need to be 9 cùn. Since Master Zhāng expressed this theory, the doctors nowadays all follow it.

愚嘗聞當世談經絡者言：自缺盆中天突至歧骨之推端九寸；自歧骨至臍中八寸；自臍中至橫骨上廉五寸云。此豈經之本意乎？

I have heard people nowadays discussing the channels and network vessels, saying that:

- It is 9 cùn from Tiān Tū (Rèn 22) at Quē Pén (the supraclavicular fossa) to the end of Qí Gǔ (the bone junction).
- It is 8 cùn from Qí Gǔ to the center of umbilicus.
- It is 5 cùn from the center of umbilicus to the upper border of Héng Gǔ (the transverse bone).

How can these be the original meaning of the Classic?

按：皇甫氏王氏滑氏之輩皆云：自缺盆中天突至髑骬九寸，髑骬至臍中八寸，臍中至橫骨六寸半是經意也。

Comments: Master Huángfǔ Mì, Master Wáng Bīng[41] and Master Huá Bórén all said:

- It is 9 cùn from Tiān Tū (Rèn 22) at Quē Pén (the supraclavicular fossa) to Hé Yú (the xiphoid process).
- It is 8 cùn from Hé Yú to the center of umbilicus.
- It is 6.5 cùn from the center of umbilicus to the upper border of Héng Gǔ (the transverse bone).

---

41. Wáng Bīng 王冰 (710-805) was a *Táng* dynasty doctor and the author of *Cì Zhù Huáng Dì Sù Wèn* 《次注黃帝素問》 (Annotation on Plain Questions of the Yellow Emperor), published in 762.

These are the meaning of the Classic.

予不才，雖不足以論先學之是非，唯恨張氏背經旨，且差四
子之說而立異說，誤骨度也。予是以論先輩之是非，以示同
志之者。詳議如左。

My humble opinion is that even though I am unqualified to discuss the correctness or incorrectness of previous scholars,[42] I only regret that Master Zhāng Jièbīn turned away from the meaning in the Classic and set up divergent theories from the other four scholars,[43] misunderstanding standard bone measurement. Therefore, I discuss the correctness or incorrectness of the previous scholars to show that I am of a similar mind [with the four scholars].

For detailed discussion, see below.

42. In East Asian culture, even strong opinions were often expressed with humility. The reader should not mistake this for doubt in the mind of the author.
43. The *four scholars* probably refers to Huángfǔ Mì, Wáng Bīng, Huá Bórén, and Gāo Wǔ 高武, who is mentioned below.

三

Chapter 3

胸腹之骨度，遠世所以誤者，熟考之十四經發揮。任脈伯仁
氏曰：靈樞經曰：髑骬（即歧骨也）以下至天樞（天樞，足
陽明經之穴，臍旁二寸，蓋臍與平直也）長八寸，而中脘居
中是也。然人胃有大小，不可拘以身寸，但髑骬至臍中，以
八寸為度，各依部分取之云。

As to why generations of the distant past made mistakes regarding standard
bone measurement on the chest and abdomen, one should check *Shí Sì Jīng Fā
Huī*[44] carefully. In the Rèn vessel section, Master Huá Bórén said:

> *Líng Shū Jīng*[45] says: "From Hé Yú (meaning the bone junction - Qí
> Gǔ)[46] down to Tiān Shū (ST 25) (Tiān Shū is a point of the foot yáng-
> míng channel; it is 2 cùn lateral to the umbilicus, and is level with the
> umbilicus) is 8 cùn in length," and Zhōng Wǎn (Rèn 12) resides in the
> middle. However, people have larger or smaller stomachs, so one cannot
> be inflexible when using body-cùn. Still, from Hé Yú to the center of the
> umbilicus, use 8 cùn as the measurement; depend on these divisions of
> the region in each [person] to find it.

夫惟伯仁發揮經旨，周悉詳盡，反復丁寧。既如此，後人學
經絡者，莫不依之，誠為經絡之學則矣。

Only Huá Bórén elaborated on the meaning of the Classic thoroughly and
comprehensively, with repeated exhortations. Thus, later generations learning

---

44. *Shí Sì Jīng Fā Huī*《十四經發揮》(Elaboration on the Fourteen Channels) was written by Huá Shòu 滑壽 (1341, *Yuán*). Huá Shòu is also known as
Huá Bórén 滑伯仁.
45. In *Líng Shū • Gǔ Dù*, Chapter 14.
46. The author is confident that Hé Yú refers to the xiphoid process, but here
the note in *Shí Sì Jīng Fā Huī* says it means Qí Gǔ (bone junction 歧骨). He
explains his dismissal of that below.

the channels and network vessels should follow this; it really is the standard of the channel theory.

張氏以歧骨分骨度，其意蓋（即歧骨也）本於如此之細註
歟。然則不達經所謂髑骭之義也。

Master Zhāng Jièbīn used Qí Gǔ (the bone junction) to divide the standard bone measurement; his idea was rooted in "(meaning the bone junction - Qí Gǔ)" from this detailed annotation [by Huá Bórén].[47] However, he did not have insight into the meaning of Hé Yú (the xiphoid process) in the Classic.

愚按：「即歧骨也」之細註，好事者所加也乎。或歧字，蔽
字之誤歟。伯仁之才，何有髑骭、蔽骨、歧骨之義不明歟？
即歧骨也者，非伯仁之言也，必矣。何以言之？「所謂人胃
有大小，不可拘以身寸，但髑骭至臍中以八寸為度，各依部
分取之云」，以此為證，伯仁如此叮嚀而誘人也。然今諸
家多以歧骨分骨度，豈可乎！經曰：缺盆至髑骭九寸。如其
至歧骨有九寸，則經直可說至歧骨，何言之髑骭哉？依文原
義，經意可觀也。嗚呼甚哉，諸家之誤也！尚為初學作詳解
如左。

I humbly comment: The detailed annotation "meaning Qí Gǔ (the bone junction)" must have been added by some officious person. Perhaps the word *junction* (qí 歧) was a mistake for *covering* (bì 蔽).[48] Regarding the ability of Huá Bórén, how could the meaning of Hé Yú (xiphoid process), Bì Gǔ (the covering bone), and Qí Gǔ (bone junction) be unclear to him? "Meaning Qí Gǔ (the bone junction)" must certainly not be the words of Huá Bórén![49] Why do I say that? "However, people have larger or smaller stomachs, so one cannot be inflexible when using body-cùn. Still, from Hé Yú (the xiphoid process) to

47. Note that Huá Bórén's book was published almost 300 years before Zhāng Jièbīn's books, and Zhāng surely used it as a reference.
48. *Bì Gǔ* (covering bone) is another name for the xiphoid process. So if *Qí Gǔ* 歧骨 (the bone junction) was mistakenly written for *Bì Gǔ* 蔽骨 (xiphoid process), everything would be in agreement.
49. The author means some later editor must have inserted these words. He does not believe they were written by Huá Bórén himself.

the center of the umbilicus, use 8 cùn as the measurement; depend on these divisions of the region in each [person] to find it." This is the proof; Huá Bórén exhorted repeatedly, trying to guide people.

However, scholars today all use Qí Gǔ (the bone junction) to divide standard bone measurement; how can this be?!

The Classic says: It is 9 cùn from Quē Pén (the supraclavicular fossa) to Hé Yú (the xiphoid process). If it is 9 cùn from [Quē Pén] to Qí Gǔ (the bone junction), the Classic could have directly said Qí Gǔ; why did it need to say Hé Yú?

The idea of the Classic can be found in the original meaning of the text.

Alas! All the scholars have misunderstood! I have made a thorough explanation below for beginners.

Chapter 4

經曰：缺盆至䯏骬九寸度之者，先上定天突又定兩乳間於膻中，而自天突至膻中量之，為六寸八分也。言天突下一寸璇璣，璇璣下一寸華蓋，華蓋下一寸六分紫宮，紫宮下一寸六分玉堂，玉堂下一寸六分膻中也，合六寸八分也。

The Classic says: "It is 9 cùn from Quē Pén (the supraclavicular fossa) to Hé Yú (the xiphoid process)," so locate Tiān Tū (Rèn 22)[50] on the top first and then locate Dàn Zhōng (Rèn 17) between the nipples. The measurement from Tiān Tū (Rèn 22) to Dàn Zhōng (Rèn 17) is 6.8 cùn.

- Xuán Jī (Rèn 21) is 1 cùn below Tiān Tū (Rèn 22).
- Huá Gài (Rèn 20) is 1 cùn below Xuán Jī (Rèn 21).
- Zǐ Gōng (Rèn 19) is 1.6 cùn below Huá Gài (Rèn 20).
- Yù Táng (Rèn 18) is 1.6 cùn below Zǐ Gōng (Rèn 19).
- Dàn Zhōng (Rèn 17) is 1.6 cùn below Yù Táng (Rèn 18).

The above total is 6.8 cùn.

又膻中下一寸六分之處，當為中庭穴也（當於歧骨上際，此寸用上六寸八分之一寸六分）。又中庭下六分之處當為䯏骬之端也（䯏骬一名蔽骨，一名尾翳，又謂鳩尾骨，蔽心骨也）。上自天突下䯏骬，通而度之，即有九寸，此非予臆說也，經所謂缺盆至䯏骬九寸者是也。

Zhōng Tíng (Rèn 16) is at the site 1.6 cùn below Dàn Zhōng (Rèn 17). (It should be on the upper border of Qí Gǔ (the bone junction); use [the equivalent of] 1.6 cùn out of the 6.8 cùn above).

The tip of Hé Yú (the xiphoid process) is 6 fēn below Zhōng Tíng (Rèn 16). (Hé Yú is also named Bì Gǔ (*the covering bone*); other names are Jiū Wěi Gǔ (*turtledove tail bone*) and Bì Xīn Gǔ (*heart-covering bone*)).

---

50. The author considers Quē Pén (the supraclavicular fossa) and Tiān Tū (Rèn 22) to be at the same level horizontally.

When measuring, it is 9 cùn altogether from Tiān Tū (Rèn 22) down to Hé Yú (the xiphoid process). This is not my assumption; the Classic says that it is 9 cùn from Quē Pén (the supraclavicular fossa) to Hé Yú.

經分骨度，皆以用其處之界限也。假令天樞至橫骨，肘至腕之類也。聖人之言不苟。

The Classic divides up standard bone measurement by using boundaries of certain areas, for example, from Tiān Shū (ST 25) to Héng Gǔ (the transverse bone), from the elbow to the wrist, and so forth. The words of the sages are very conscientious.

夫髑骬者，蔽心骨，而從歧骨之間垂下，如指大骨也，附於胸骨之部分也，是胸腹之限也。經至髑骬分骨度，豈不宜乎是為胸腹之界限也！不察於此而以歧骨為限，以分骨度，豈合經旨乎！捨蔽骨而操歧骨，豈和骨度乎！故余不隨當世之說也，是以今為骨度正誤之圖，以示友人。

Hé Yú (the xiphoid process) means the heart covering bone (Bì Gǔ); it hangs down from Qí Gǔ (the bone junction) like a large finger bone. It attaches to part of the sternum and is the boundary between the chest and abdomen. The Classic divides standard bone measurement at Hé Yú; isn't this an appropriate boundary between the chest and abdomen?! If this is not understood, and Qí Gǔ is used as the border to divide standard bone measurement, how can it match the meaning of the Classic?! If Bì Gǔ (the covering bone) is ignored and Qí Gǔ is followed, how could it match standard bone measurement?!

So I do not follow what modern people say, and wrote *Correcting Errors in Standard Bone Measurement with Illustrations* to show this to my friends.

蓋雖胸腹之骨度，以蔽骨為界限，而蔽骨由人不見或有浮沉長短異。不拘之，只從天突至中庭八寸四分，胸部直寸法皆可用之矣。蓋中庭當歧骨之上一分許也（一說云，中庭，歧骨之上六分；膻中，歧骨之上二寸二分云；又云：胸部直骨

度，天突至歧骨，可為九寸云，此甚誤也！如所謂，則胸部
之寸方皆差，故有害也必矣 ）。

Even though Bì Gǔ (the covering bone) is the border for standard bone
measurement on the chest and abdomen, it cannot be seen and there are differences in its depth and length. Do not stick to it rigidly; just follow 8.4 cùn
[as the distance] from Tiān Tū (Rèn 22) to Zhōng Tíng (Rèn 16). This can be
used for the vertical body-cùn method on the chest.

Zhōng Tíng (Rèn 16) is approximately 1 fēn above Qí Gǔ (the bone junction).
(Another theory is that Zhōng Tíng (Rèn 16) is 6 fēn above Qí Gǔ and Dàn
Zhōng (Rèn 17) is 2.2 cùn above Qí Gǔ. This theory also says that the vertical
standard bone measurement on the chest from Tiān Tū (Rèn 22) to Qí Gǔ
can be considered 9 cùn. This is so wrong! If one follows that, the cùn measurement on the chest region will be wrong, so it will certainly come to harm!).

按：從歧骨際下長一寸當為髑骬之分，而從歧骨際至臍中當
為九寸，大腹直寸法用之矣 。是非予臆說，詳議口授 。

Comments: The portion of Hé Yú (the xiphoid process) from the border of Qí
Gǔ (the bone junction) downward should be considered 1 cùn long.[51] From
the border of Qí Gǔ to the center of the umbilicus is 9 cùn, which should be
used for the vertical body-cùn method on the abdomen.[52]

This is not my assumption; I have discussed it in detail and give oral instructions.

---

51. Above, the author stated that the xiphoid is 0.6 cùn. Here he says 1 cùn
long. Unless he was rounding it off to a more user-friendly number, the reason
for this discrepancy is puzzling.
52. Since the tip of the xiphoid may be hard to feel, the author says on a practi-
cal level to consider the xiphoid process 1 cùn long. Then you can call the
distance from the bone junction to the center of the umbilicus 9 cùn. This is
easier for the practitioner than using 8 cùn from the tip of the xiphoid process
to the center of umbilicus.

巨闕一穴，今人多言臍上六寸，非也，是亦自張氏始。是由
歧骨蔽骨之差也，當為六寸五分矣。

Jù Què (Rèn 14): Nowadays people say it is 6 cùn above the umbilicus; this
is wrong and is also from Master Zhāng Jièbīn. This is because of the mistake
regarding Qí Gǔ (the bone junction) and Bì Gǔ (the covering bone). It should
be 6.5 cùn.

伯仁曰：上脘在巨闕下一寸五分，去蔽骨三寸。巨闕在鳩尾
下一寸，鳩尾在蔽骨端，其骨垂下如鳩形，故以為名，臆前
蔽骨下五分（鳩尾穴也）。人無蔽骨者，從歧骨際下一寸（
蔽骨之長）。

Huá Bórén said: Shàng Wǎn (Rèn 13) is located 1.5 cùn below Jù Què (Rèn
14) and 3 cùn from Bì Gǔ (the covering bone). Jù Què (Rèn 14) is located 1
cùn below Jiū Wěi (Rèn 15). Jiū Wěi (Rèn 15) is located at the end of Bì Gǔ;
the bone hangs down in the shape of a turtledove, so Jiū Wěi (*turtledove tail*) is
taken as the point name. It is 5 fēn below Bì Gǔ on the anterior chest (meaning
the Jiū Wěi (Rèn 15) point); in people who do not have Bì Gǔ, [this point is] 1
cùn below the border of Qí Gǔ (the bone junction) [the length of the covering
bone].

愚謂骨度之法，自骬骬至臍中八寸，上脘當於臍上五寸，去
蔽骨三寸也。巨闕在蔽骨下一寸五分，巨闕與上脘相去一寸
五分也。須知，巨闕臍上六寸五分也。

I humbly say: The method for standard bone measurement is that it is 8 cùn
from Hé Yú (the xiphoid process) to the center of the umbilicus.

- Shàng Wǎn (Rèn 13) is located 5 cùn above the umbilicus, 3 cùn from Bì Gǔ (the covering bone).
- Jù Què (Rèn 14) is located 1.5 cùn below Bì Gǔ.
- The distance between Jù Què (Rèn 14) and Shàng Wǎn (Rèn 13) is 1.5 cùn.

People should know that Jù Què (Rèn 14) is located 6.5 cùn above the umbilicus.

近年，岡本為竹著十四經和語鈔，任脈巨闕上脘說云：滑氏巨闕註誤。愚謂伯仁之註全不誤，巨闕上脘之和語之說全誤也。學者宜審之。

Recently, Gāngběn Wéizhú wrote *Shí Sì Jīng Hé Yǔ Chāo.*[53] Regarding Jù Què (Rèn 14) and Shàng Wǎn (Rèn 13) on the Rèn vessel, it says: "The annotation of Master Huá on Jù Què (Rèn 14) was wrong." I say that the annotation of Huá Bórén was not wrong at all. The theory on Jù Què (Rèn 14) and Shàng Wǎn (Rèn 13) in *Shí Sì Jīng Hé Yǔ Chāo* is completely wrong. Scholars should check this carefully.

---

53. Gāngběn Wéizhú 岡本為竹 was also was known as Gāngběn Yībào 岡本一抱 (Jp: Okamoto, Ippō) (1654-1716). He was a renowned doctor and author in Japan with 23 publications. *Shí Sì Jīng Hé Yǔ Chāo*《十四經和語鈔》(Jp: *Jyū Shi Kei Wa Go Shō*) (The Fourteen Channels in Japanese) was published in the sixth year of Yuán Lù's (Gēn Roku) reign 元禄 (1693).

經曰：臍至橫骨六寸半矣。張氏云，自臍心至毛際曲骨穴折
五寸，臍下骨度等用之。今人多從之。按，臍下骨度不可等
為五寸也，等取於五寸者，非也。蓋任脈與腎經者，取臍下
於五寸而已，非為骨度也。

The Classic says: It is 6.5 cùn from the umbilicus to Héng Gǔ (the transverse
bone). Master Zhāng Jièbīn said: From the center of the umbilicus to Qū Gǔ
(Rèn 2) in the hairy region is equivalent to 5 cùn; use this as the standard bone
measurement below the umbilicus. Nowadays everybody follows this.

Comments: The standard bone measurement below the umbilicus cannot be
equivalent to 5 cùn; finding points using 5 cùn will be wrong. On the Rèn vessel and kidney channel, we can use a distance of 5 cùn below the umbilicus, but
it is not the standard bone measurement [for the whole region].

度之者，先取神闕與曲骨中間之長，折作五，即折出四而伸
之，當於神闕與曲骨，則上端神闕，下端曲骨也，每中折點
之也，中極、關元、石門、陰交也，通而為五寸，氣海一穴
在石門與陰交中間也。

[Use a length of straw or string to] measure the distance between Shén Què
(Rèn 8) and Qū Gǔ (Rèn 2). Fold it into fifths, meaning fold [the string] four
times; then unfold it and place it between Shén Què (Rèn 8) and Qū Gǔ (Rèn
2).[54] Thus, the upper point is Shén Què (Rèn 8) and the lower point is Qū Gǔ
(Rèn 2). Then locate the points at the middle of each fold to get Zhōng Jí (Rèn

---

54. Since there are 5 cùn between the umbilicus and the upper border of the
pubic bone on the Rèn vessel, folding the straw or string four times to make
five equal portions will give the individual's body cùn measurement for this
region. It is not easy to fold a string into fifths; one may need to re-adjust the
folds until there are five equal portions.

3), Guān Yuán (Rèn 4), Shí Mén (Rèn 5), and Yīn Jīao (Rèn 7) for the 5 cùn in total. Qì Hǎi (Rèn 6) is between Shí Mén (Rèn 5) and Yīn Jīao (Rèn 7).

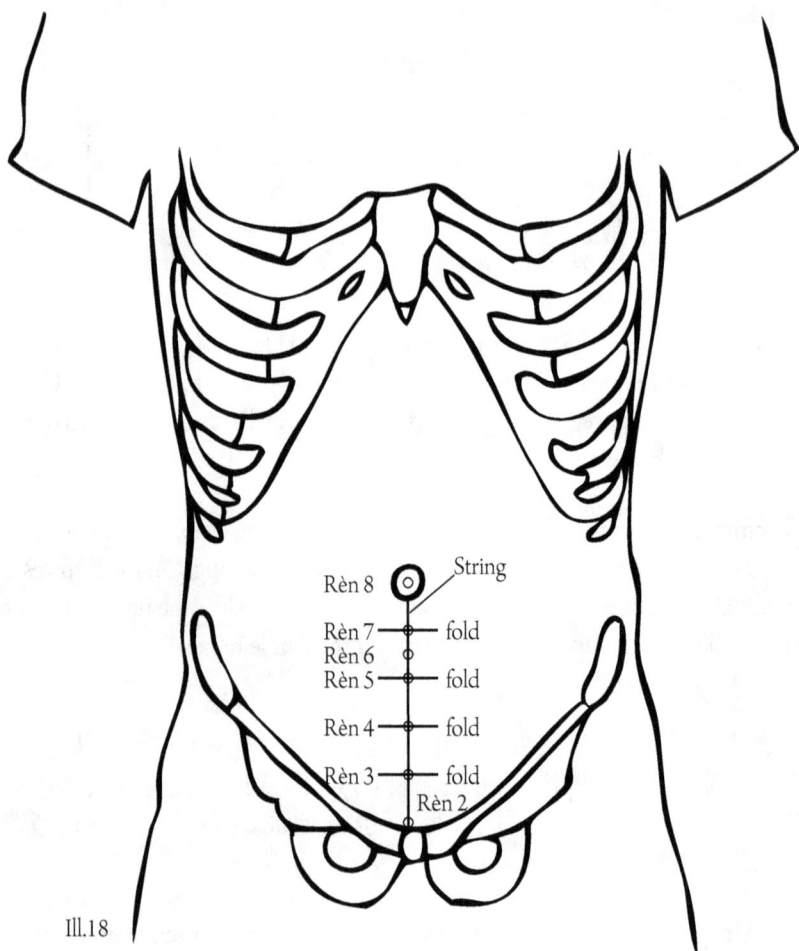

Ill.18

腎經亦如此：自橫骨至肓俞，折作五，可量也 。

It is the same for the kidney channel: Measure from Héng Gǔ (the transverse bone) to Huāng Shù (KI 16) [with a piece of straw or string] and fold it into fifths.[55]

---

55. This would be used to find Héng Gǔ (KI 11), Dà Hè (KI 12), Qì Xué (KI 13), Sì Mǎn (KI 14), Zhōng Zhù (KI 15), and Huāng Shù (KI 16).

脾胃之兩經者，可取臍下於六寸半矣。等取於五寸，則胃經
氣來低而不居本位也。學者宜校正焉。經曰：臍至橫骨六寸
半者非歟。今言五寸者，是歟。其如之何，有圖，見前。

The spleen and stomach channels below the umbilicus can be measured as 6.5
cùn. If they were equal to the 5 cùn [of the Rèn vessel and kidney channel], Guī
Lái (ST 29)[56] on the stomach channel would be lower and not in its original
position. Scholars should proofread and correct this. The Classic says [in *Gŭ
Dù Piān*]: From the umbilicus to Héng Gŭ (the transverse bone) is 6.5 cùn,
but this is wrong. Today's theory of 5 cùn is correct. What this looks like can be
found in the previous diagrams.[57]

---

56. Guī Lái 歸來 (ST 29): The original text has the character qì lái 氣來 instead of guī lái 歸來; this has been changed based on the correct name for the
point. This error occurs once more in the text below.
57. Please refer to the two earlier diagrams and text on pages 35 and 36. In the
diagram that the author endorses, Guī Lái (ST 29) is on the upper border of the
pubic bone and Qì Chōng (ST 30) is on the lower border of the pubic bone.
Because the six points on the stomach channel from Tiān Shū (ST 25) to Qì
Chōng (ST 30) finish *below* the pubic bone, they are not directly lateral to the
six points of the kidney channel from Huāng Shù (KI 16) down to Héng Gŭ
(KI 11) which finish on the *upper* border of the pubic bone. This extra length
to reach the bottom of the pubic bone makes 6.5 cùn rather than 5 cùn. The 5
cùn measurement we use today for the length below the umbilicus is not found
in *Gŭ Dù Piān*, so the author feels that the Classic has an error.

Chapter 7

經曰：兩乳闊九寸半，是骨度也。圖翼曰：灸法以八寸為當。今醫有謂張氏發明者，殊不知焉，明於滑氏發揮也，豈是張氏之發明乎！兩乳八寸不知所以然者多焉。愚謂：自膻中橫至神封二寸，神封至乳中二寸，左右合而得八寸。施鍼灸於胸腹者，橫開之寸法依之矣。

The Classic says: The width between the nipples is 9.5 cùn; this is the standard bone measurement. *Tú Yì* says: It is appropriate to use 8 cùn when applying moxibustion.

Nowadays doctors say this was invented by Master Zhāng Jièbīn. Little do they realize that it was elaborated on and clarified by Master Huá Bórén, so how can it be Master Zhāng's invention?! Lots of people do not know why the width between the nipples is 8 cùn.

My comments: It is 2 cùn horizontally from Dàn Zhōng (Rèn 17) to Shén Fēng (KI 23); it is 2 cùn from Shén Fēng (KI 23) to Rǔ Zhōng (ST 17); it is 8 cùn in total from the left to the right side. When applying acupuncture and moxibustion on the chest and abdomen, this transverse body-cùn measurement should be followed.

八
Chapter 8

經曰：肩至肘一尺七寸。張氏云：肩者，肩端也。愚按：肩端自肩髃至肘曲池為一尺七寸歟也，是亦非也。近年世醫多宗之是之，且樓英說共合，而施於世。如此則可謂以誤傳誤矣。一人誤而眾人誤焉，可嘆之甚。

The Classic says: It is 1.7 chǐ from the shoulder to the elbow. Master Zhāng said: *Shoulder* means the end of the shoulder.

My comments: It is incorrect that there are 1.7 chǐ from Jiān Yú (LI 15) at the end of the shoulder to Qū Chí (LI 11) on the elbow. Doctors today all follow this, and Lóu Yīng also agreed with this theory and imposed it on the world. Thus, this is what is called "passing on a mistake because of a mistake." One person is wrong and then everyone is wrong. Sigh!

夫以骨度篇所說人長七尺五寸者，橫直等謂也。如張氏之說，自肩端量，則中乎脊骨而相捨兩肩之間，惡合骨度乎！可謂張氏千慮之失也。介賓既如此，況後學于？

Using what *Gǔ Dù Piān* says, the human body is 7.5 chǐ tall and the transverse and vertical measurements are equivalent.[58] According to Master Zhāng, it is measured from the end of the shoulder. The center is [actually] on the spine, but he ignores the space between both shoulders.[59] This does not agree with

---

58. This means that the height of the human body is the same as the distance between the tips of the middle fingers when the arms are extended and level with the shoulders.

59. *Nèi Jīng* says that it is 1.7 chǐ from the shoulder to the elbow. The question is, where on the shoulder is this measurement taken? Zhāng said it is from the Jiān Yú (LI 15) region, but the author disagrees. He felt it was from the spine, at Dà Zhuì (Dū 14). *Gǔ Dù Piān* says it is 1.7 chǐ from the shoulder to the elbow, 1.25 chǐ from the elbow to the wrist, 4 cùn from the wrist to the base joint of the middle finger, and 4.5 cùn from the base joint to the end of the middle

the standard bone measurement! Master Zhāng was wise but he was not free from errors. If [Zhāng] Jièbīn was like this, what about later scholars?![60]

九

Chapter 9

按：肩至肘一尺七寸度之者，舉臂伸手於左右，而自大椎下
脊中至肘尖可為一尺七寸也。今人肩端肩髃至曲池為一尺七
寸者繆也。

Comments: For the 1.7 chǐ measurement from the shoulder to the elbow, lift the arm and extend the hands out to the sides. From the center of the spine below Dà Zhuī (Dū 14) to the tip of the elbow is 1.7 chǐ.

Nowadays people say that it is 1.7 chǐ from the Jiān Yú (LI 15) at end of the shoulder to Qū Chí (LI 11); this is wrong.

十

Chapter 10

經曰：中指本節至末四寸半也。愚私按：半之一字衍文，削
去可也。不然不合於骨度也。（ 尚口授 ）

---

finger. This adds up to 3.8 chǐ on one side; taking both sides into account, the total is 7.6 chǐ from the tip of one middle finger to the other. If the human body is 7.5 chǐ tall and the transverse and vertical measurements are equivalent, the total more or less agrees. (In Chapter 10, the author commented that the length from the base joint to the end of the middle finger should be 4 cùn not 4.5 cùn. If this number is used, the total width from finger to finger will be exactly 7.5 chǐ.) If instead, the 1.7 chǐ length from the shoulder to the elbow is taken from the Jiān Yú (LI 15) region, there would be additional cùn from the Jiān Yú (LI 15) region to the spine, making the grand total of 7.5 chǐ wrong.

60. The text has *yú* 于 when it should be *hū* 乎. However, this is an 'empty word' here and makes no difference to the English reader.

The Classic says: It is 4.5 cùn from the base joint to the tip of the middle finger.

My personal comments: The word 0.5 (half, *bàn* 半) is extra and can be removed. Otherwise, it does not match standard bone measurement.[61] (There are further oral instructions.)

十一

Chapter 11

胃經下行腹者，考之於經· 氣府論曰：挾鳩尾之外，當乳下三寸，挾胃脘各五；挾臍廣三寸各三；下臍二寸挾之各三云云。經文浩浩乎如望洋，因而諸說亦不同也。

Regarding the stomach channel which descends the abdomen, when checking *Qì Fǔ Lùn*[62] of the Classic, it says: "There are five points located [on the line] 3 cùn lateral to Jiū Wěi (Rèn 15), below the nipples and lateral to stomach duct. There are three points located [on the same line that is] 3 cùn lateral to the umbilicus. [Starting] 2 cùn below the umbilicus, there are three bilateral points," and so forth. The text of the Classic is as expansive as the ocean, therefore various theories are different.

甲乙經曰：腹自不容至氣衝二十四穴，挾幽門兩旁各一寸五分。張氏從之。

Jiǎ Yǐ Jīng[63] says: From Bù Róng (ST 19) to Qì Chōng (ST 30) on the abdomen, 24 points[64] are located 1.5 cùn lateral to Yōu Mén (KI 21). Master Zhāng Jièbīn agreed.

---

61. For the reason, see the footnote in Chapter 8.
62. This refers to *Sù Wèn* 《 素問 》, Chapter 59.
63. *Jiǎ Yǐ Jīng* 《 甲乙經 》, also named *Zhēn Jiǔ Jiǎ Yǐ Jīng* 《 針灸甲乙經 》 (The Systematic Classic of Acupuncture and Moxibustion), was written by Huángfǔ Mì 皇甫謐 (282 C.E., *Jìn* dynasty).
64. 24 points means 12 bilateral points.

發揮註曰：自不容至滑肉門，去中行各三寸；自天樞至氣來去中行各二寸。馬氏從之，高武亦同之，李梴異焉。愚今去中行以二寸為是也。

An annotation in *Fā Huī* says: [The channel] is 3 cùn to each side of the midline from Bù Róng (ST 19) to Huá Ròu Mén (ST 24). It is 2 cùn to each side of the midline from Tiān Shū (ST 25) to Guī Lái (ST 29).[65] Master Mǎ Shí[66] and Gāo Wǔ[67] agreed, but Lǐ Chān[68] disagreed. I now think this [all] should be 2 cùn lateral to the midline.

按：不容非幽門旁也。先輩謂幽門旁對巨闕者，非也，不合於骨度也。骨度之法，自鮚骭之端至臍中八寸用豎，兩乳之間八寸用橫也。人無鮚骭者，歧骨至臍中至九寸而可度也。以此法，巨闕為臍上六寸五分；幽門者，巨闕旁；不容者，可為天樞上六寸矣。

Comments: Bù Róng (ST 19) is not lateral to Yōu Mén (KI 21). Anyone from the previous generations who said it is lateral to Yōu Mén (KI 21) and opposite Jù Què (Rèn 14) is wrong; this does not match standard bone measurement. In the standard bone measurement method, it is 8 cùn from the end of Hé Yú (the xiphoid process) vertically to the center of the umbilicus; the horizontal distance between the nipples is 8 cùn. In people who do not have Hé Yú, it is 9 cùn from Qí Gǔ (the bone junction) to the center of the umbilicus and this can

---

65. Guī Lái 歸來 (ST 29): The original text has the characters *qì lái* 氣來 instead of *guī lái* 歸來; this has been changed based on the correct name for the point.

66. Master Mǎ refers to Mǎ Shí 馬蒔, a doctor of the *Míng* dynasty and the author of *Huáng Dì Nèi Jīng Sù Wèn Zhù Zhèng Fā Wēi*《黃帝內經素問注證發微》(Annotation, Affirmation and Elaboration on Plain Question in Yellow Emperor's Inner Classic) and *Huáng Dì Nèi Jīng Líng Shū Zhù Zhèng Fā Wēi*《黃帝內經靈樞注證發微》(Annotation, Affirmation, and Elaboration on Magic Pivot in Yellow Emperor's Inner Classic).

67. Gāo Wǔ 高武 was a *Míng* dynasty doctor. He was the author of *Zhēn Jiǔ Jù Yīng*《針灸聚英》(Gathered Blooms of Acupuncture and Moxibustion), published in 1529.

68. Lǐ Chān 李梴 was another *Míng* dynasty doctor. He was the author of *Yī Xué Rù Mén*《醫學入門》(The Gateway to Medicine), published in 1575.

be measured. When using this method, Jù Què (Rèn 14) is 6.5 cùn above the umbilicus; Yōu Mén (KI 21) is lateral to Jù Què (Rèn 14); but Bù Róng (ST 19) is located 6 cùn above Tiān Shū (ST 25).[69]

胃經下行腹者，自不容至歸來去任中各二寸也 。

For the stomach channel, the points from Bù Róng (ST 19) descending the abdomen to Guī Lái (ST 29) are located 2 cùn lateral to the Rèn vessel on the midline.

○十四經曰：日月，期門下五分 。愚按，非也，當為一寸五分 。

Shí Sì Jīng says: Rì Yuè (GB 24) is located 5 fēn below Qī Mén (LV 14). My comment: This is wrong; it should be 1.5 cùn [below Qí Mén (LV 14)].

○溫溜穴（ 口傳 ）。

Wēn Liū (LI 7): (oral instructions).

○小腸經肩貞 、臑俞 、天宗 、秉風 、曲垣，經行穴處（ 口傳 ）

On the small intestine channel, Jiān Zhēn (SI 9), Nào Shù (SI 10), Tiān Zōng (SI 11), Bǐng Fēng (SI 12), and Qū Yuàn (SI 13): these points are located on the line of the channel (oral instructions).

---

69. The author feels that Jù Què (Rèn 14) and Yōu Mén (KI 21) are 6.5 cùn above the umbilicus but Bù Róng (ST 19) is located 6 cùn above the umbilicus, so Bù Róng (ST 19) cannot be level with the other two points. The reason for this is that by the written description of the location, Jù Què (Rèn 14) is located by counting from the top down and the discrepancy between the bone junction and the xiphoid process makes a difference in this (see Chapter 5). Yōu Mén (KI 21) is defined as being lateral to Jù Què (Rèn 14) so it is at the same level. But Bù Róng (ST 19) is defined as being 6 cùn above the umbilicus, so it is not level with the other two.

○髀關二穴（口傳）

Bì Guān (ST 31), bilateral point (oral instructions).

此四章著於俞穴辨解

These four items were written in *Shù Xuè Biàn Jie*.[70]

十二

Chapter 12

督脈之穴處，張景岳定於脊節之高處者，非也，豈然乎？
按：周身之俞穴者，所為榮衛神氣之游行交會而皆孔隙也，
故處在或大骨之際，小骨之下；大筋之下，小筋之上；或骨
際陷中空隙也。一不在尖角之骨上，所無孔隙，故曰孔穴
焉。如張氏說，豈節上所無孔隙而榮衛神氣之會者也哉！須
為千慮之失矣。余斷然而不從。學者察焉。滑氏取於脊骨之
低處者是也。

Zhāng Jǐngyuè located points of the Dū vessel at the highest place on the vertebrae. Why is this wrong?

Comments: Points all over the body are the holes where *yíng*-construction,
wèi-defense, and *shén*-spirit qì flow and meet, so they should be located either
on the border of a big bone, below a small bone, below a big sinew, above a
small sinew, or in a depression along the border of a bone. Not one is on the tip

70. *Shù Xuè Biàn Jie* 《俞穴辨解》 (Jp: *Yu Ketsu Ben Kai*) (Differentiation
and Analysis of Points) was written by the same author, Cùnshàng Zōngzhàn
村上宗占 (Jp: Sōsen Murakami), and published in 1754. The *four items* refers
to the short text above regarding Rì Yuè (GB 24), Wēn Liū (LI 7), the points
on the small intestine channel, and Bì Guān (ST 31). More detail is in this
other book, and the author intended to give oral instructions to his apprentices,
either to keep some of his teachings more secret, or because it was easier to
show them than to describe it in writing.

or corner of a bone where there is no small opening; this is why they are called *holes*.[71] If it were as Master Zhāng said, how could *yíng*, *wèi*, and *shén* qì flow and meet when there is no hole in the vertebra! This must be a rare mistake made by the wise. I absolutely will not follow this. Scholars should scrutinize this. Master Huá Bórén correctly located points at the low places on the spine.

十三

Chapter 13

背俞寸方辨不同

Differentiation of Cùn Measurement for the Back Transport Points

膀胱經背二行。滑伯仁曰：相去脊中為一寸半，三行相去脊中為三寸也。張介賓曰：在二行當為二寸，在三行當為三寸半云也。二氏之說，各不同。蓋滑氏為是，張氏為非。雖近世之人謂滑氏為是，或張氏為非，而未知其是非之本源者多焉。知其本源而後可謂是非也。

The second line on the back is the urinary bladder channel.[72] Huá Bórén said: It is 1.5 cùn from the center of the spine and the third line is 3.0 cùn from the center of the spine. Zhāng Jiebīn said: The second line is 2.0 cùn [from the center of the spine] and the third line should be 3.5 cùn [from the center of the spine]. The theories of those two masters disagree. Master Huá is correct and Master Zhāng is wrong. Though people today say that Master Huá was correct and Master Zhāng was wrong, many do not know the original source for [the determination of] incorrect or correct. People should know the original source before they can discuss whether it is incorrect or correct.

---

71. The English reader should note that the character for point (*xué* 穴) actually means a *hole* or *opening*. *Point* is not a literal translation of the character.
72. The Dū vessel is the first line of the back. The inner urinary bladder channel line is the second. The outer urinary bladder channel line is the third.

夫惟背二行，五藏俞穴者，出於背俞，形志二篇矣。伯仁觀
經旨也，詳而正矣，誠為經絡之達人矣。雖不見其人，視十
四經發揮，則思過半矣。介賓者，天行聰明無不通於諸家，
而博識精敏也，註於內經也，啟蘊奧而大有助於醫家者也。
我視其類經，則起而再拜，稽首而讀焉。嗟呼！非常之人，
可以讚焉，可以賞焉，然於背俞之寸法也，誤者何乎也，蓋
千慮一失也。

The second line on the back is where the transport points of five *zàng*-organs
are located; this is from two chapters [of the Classic]: *Bèi Shù* and *Xíng Zhì*. Huá
Bórén checked the meaning of the Classic thoroughly and was correct. He
indeed was a well-informed person regarding the channels and network vessels. Even though I never met him, when I read *Shí Sì Jīng Fā Huī*, I understood
a lot. Zhāng Jièbīn was intelligent and understood all the schools and theories;
he was learned and alert. He annotated *Nèi Jīng*, explored its hidden secrets, and
greatly benefited medical doctors. When I read his *Lèi Jīng*, I got up and bowed
twice, kowtowed, and read it again.

Alas! He was an extraordinary person, worthy of praise and admiration.
However, regarding the cùn-method for the back transport points, how did he
make this mistake?! This is [an example of the saying that] "even the wise make
mistakes."

靈樞·背腧篇末章曰：腎腧在十四焦之間，皆俠脊相去三寸
所云云。類註曰：此自大腧至腎腧，左右各相去脊中一寸五
分。故云：俠脊相去三寸所也。此註得經旨而正，不可改
焉。然又圖翼曰：在二行當為二寸，在三行當為三寸半云。
言出於一口而齟齬如此，可謂甚錯誤焉！所以然者，顧形志
篇草度之法，觀經意也，差矣。

Near the end of *Líng Shū· Bèi Shù*,[73] it says: Shèn Shù (UB 23) is located in the
space of the 14th vertebra [L$_2$],[74] 3 cùn away [from the same point on the other
side], embracing the spine. A note in *Lèi Jīng* says: From Dà Zhù (UB 11) to

---

73. This refers to *Líng Shū*, Chapter 51
74. According to *Jiǎ Yǐ Jīng* 《甲乙經》 and *Huáng Dì Nèi Jīng Tài Sù* 《黃
帝內經太素》, the text should have *zhuī* 椎 instead of *jiāo* 焦 here.

Shèn Shù (UB 23), the points are 1.5 cùn lateral to the spine on each side.
So, the Classic says: 3 cùn away from each other, embracing the spine. This
annotation obtained the correct meaning of the Classic; it cannot be revised.
However, *Tú Yì* says: The second line should be 2 cùn and the third line should
be 3 cùn [lateral to the midline]. These words came from the same person but
it is so wrong that they disagree like this! The reason for it is that when looking
at the straw measurement method[75] in *Xíng Zhì Piān* and reading the meaning
of the Classic, *Tú Yì* is different!

姑舉草度之經文並以張氏註文，謂其所差乎。經曰：欲知背
俞，先度其兩乳間，中折之，更以他草度去半已，即以兩隅
相柱也。

Let me give an example of straw measurement in the text of the Classic and the
annotations of Master Zhāng Jièbīn to show the discrepancy between them.
The Classic says: "If one wants to know [the location of] the back transport
points, first measure the [distance between] the nipples [with a piece of straw]
and fold it in the center. Alter another piece of straw, measuring [it to the same
length], and once half [the length of straw] is removed, use the two corners to
support each other."[76]

---

75. Straw measurement: An ancient way of locating certain points involved
taking a long piece of straw or grass, measuring one part of the body, and
using that measurement on another body part. The measured length is often
folded to find a specific proportion of that length. This was used in *Sù Wèn·
Xuè Qì Xíng Zhì Piān* and will be discussed in more detail below. Modern
people are more likely to use string than straw. This method seems to be more
popular in Japan today than in other places.
76. This is from *Sù Wèn· Xuè Qì Xíng Zhì Piān*. Essentially, one makes a triangle from two pieces of straw and uses it to locate the back transport points.
However, the description in *Sù Wèn* is ambiguous and the author disagrees
with Zhāng Jièbīn's interpretation. More explanation is given in Chapter 16.
There, he explains this passage word by word and phrase by phrase. The
translation here is based on the author's interpretation. *Xíng Zhì Piān* goes on
to give instructions on how to find all the back transport points by moving the
straw triangle down the spine. This will be discussed below.

類註曰：先以草橫量兩乳之間，中半摺折之，又另以一草
比前草而去其半，取齊中折之數，乃豎立長草，橫置短草
於下，兩頭相柱，象△三隅 。乃舉此草以量其背，令一隅居
上，齊脊中之大椎，其在下兩隅當三椎之間，即肺之俞也
云 。

A note in *Lèi Jīng* says: Use a piece of straw to measure the transverse distance
between the nipples and fold it in half at the center. Then match another piece
of straw to the length of the previous one and remove half, making it even in
length with the center fold [of the long piece]. Then put the longer piece of
straw upright and place the short straw horizontally below it. The two ends of
each straw support each other, so it is shaped like a triangle. Then use this straw
to measure the patient's back. Make the upper corner even with Dà Zhuī (Dū
14) in the center of the spine; the two lower corners will be level with the third
vertebra, which is the back transport point of the lungs.

愚按：兩乳之間為八寸也，經文先度其兩乳之間，中折之，
則一偏四寸也；更以他草度者，以另草度中折之，一偏也是
四寸也，半則二寸也，是經旨也 。

My humble comments: The distance between the nipples is 8 cùn. The text
of the Classic [says to] measure the distance between the nipples first and fold
[the straw] in half, so each segment is 4 cùn long. "Alter another piece of straw,
measuring," means [measuring] the one that is folded in half, which makes
another segment of 4 cùn. Half of that is 2 cùn, which is the meaning of the
Classic.

張氏所為者異之：先量兩乳之間，中折而又另以一草比前度
八寸之草去半，此草四寸也，以四寸之另草加八寸中折之兩
端，兩頭相柱，象△三隅云，非是，經旨無以兩隅相柱之義
矣 。以四寸之草加八寸中折之兩端也，即成三面等四寸之
象 。以之量背之俞穴，故兩穴相去四寸也 。

What Master Zhāng Jièbīn did was different: He measured the distance
between the nipples and folded the straw in half. He then used another piece

of straw to measure the previous length, which is 8 cùn long. Then he removed half, so now this piece of straw is 4 cùn long. Then he used this 4 cùn length of straw to support the two ends of the folded 8 cùn length of straw to form a tri-angle. This is not correct. This is not what Classic means by "using two corners supporting each other." Using a 4 cùn length of straw plus the two ends from the folded 8 cùn length of straw makes a 4 cùn equilateral triangle. So using his method to measure the points on the back, the distance between the points on both sides would be 4 cùn.[77]

背俞往而無不為二寸矣。背俞篇註曰：自大䐢至腎俞，左右各相去脊中一寸五分。故云：俠脊三寸所云矣。於形志篇又為四寸，如斯豈不為錯誤乎。熟按張氏背俞篇之註說，得而正矣，確乎而不可易焉然，雖草度之法誤不自覺，卻而以背俞篇之註正自己為非者歟也，斯以改而巧言穿脊骨。

Back transport points have always been [considered] 2 cùn [lateral to spine] in the past.[78] An annotation for *Bèi Shù Piān* [written by Zhāng Jièbīn] says: "From Dà Zhù (UB 11) to Shèn Shù (UB 23), each point is 1.5 cùn from the center of the spine on both sides so [*Bèi Shù Piān*] says, 'the points embrace the spine and are 3 cùn [from each other].'" However, in [Zhāng's comments on] *Xíng Zhì Piān*, the distance is 4 cùn; thus, how is it not an error!?

In Master Zhāng's annotation for *Bèi Shù Pian*, he understood and got it cor-rect. Even though he was unaware of his mistake with straw measurement, he corrected his own error with his annotations from *Bèi Shù Piān*! This is revising [the measurement] across the spine with cunning words.

---

77. This method would make the back transport points 2 cùn from the midline, not 1.5 cùn.
78. *Bèi Shù Piān* and *Xíng Zhì Piān* describe different methods for locating the back transport-points. Because of the way Zhāng interpreted *Xíng Zhì Piān*, he ended up with a distance of 4 cùn between the two sides of the inner bladder line. However, *Bèi Shù Piān* clearly states that there are 3 cùn between the two sides. So Zhāng was forced to come up with a rather convoluted argument that the spine is 1 cùn wide and that the 3 cùn of *Bèi Shù Piān* didn't count the width of the spine.

圖翼曰：脊骨內闊一寸。几（凡）云第二行俠脊一寸半，三行俠脊三寸者，除脊一寸外，淨以寸半，三寸論。故在二行當為二寸，在三行當為三寸半云。前後其言出於一口，而齟齬差謬無甚於此矣。

Tú Yì says: "[The spinous processes of] the vertebrae are 1 cùn wide. All the theories that the second line is 1.5 cùn lateral to the spine and the third line is 3 cùn lateral to the spine do not include the 1 cùn of the spine, so the net distance is 1.5 cùn [to one side] and 3 cùn [from each other]. Therefore, the second line should be 2 cùn [lateral to the midline of the spine], and the third line should be 3.5 cùn lateral."[79] The earlier and later words are from the same person, but the disagreement is nothing more than this.

張氏先誤草度之法也，經文更以他草度去半已，云此中有蘊奧而義存焉。張氏不考索之，故所為之法，象成四寸三面之象。故背之俞穴，兩穴相去為四寸也。

First Master Zhāng Jièbīn misunderstood the straw measurement method. The text of the Classic says "alter another piece of straw, measuring, and once half [of the length of straw] is removed …" This contains the secret and its meaning is preserved. Master Zhāng did not research it carefully, so the method he made resulted in a 4 cùn equilateral triangle. Thus, his back transport-points are 4 cùn away from each other.

齊之於大椎，自肺俞至脾俞下四度，則當於十三四椎而各不當於本位，豈是不為誤乎？學者以張氏所為法象量背之俞穴，試可知焉。

At the level of Dà Zhuī (Dū 14), from Fèi Shù (UB 13) down to Pí Shù (UB 20), the four measurements[80] would be level to the 13th and 14th vertebrae [L₁

---

79. This is adding in 0.5 cùn, which is the width of the spine on one side.
80. The four measurements from Fèi Shù (UB 13) down to Pí Shù (UB 20): This refers to the measurements for Fèi Shù (UB 13), Xīn Shù (UB 15), Gān Shù (UB 18), and Pí Shù (UB 20). These would be found by moving the triangle down the back. After locating Fèi Shù (UB 13) by placing the top of the triangle at Dà Zhuī (Dū 14), the top of the triangle is then placed on the spine

and L$_2$] and would not be at the level of their original position. How is this not a mistake? If scholars test the method and image made by Master Zhāng to measure the back transport points, they will know [it is wrong].

十四
Chapter 14

或曰：居古人之位，做古人之事難矣。後人議前人易焉。吾予以張氏之說數為誤者，恐不可也。張氏為天下顯名，豈得為易之乎？予應之曰：凡是為是，非為非，天下之通論也。張氏之功故不可奪焉，然期間有不合經旨者，故予辯論之舉，一廢百古人所惡，何妄意誹議乎？

Someone might say: It is difficult to live in the same conditions as the ancient people and to copy the things they did but it is easy to criticize people of previous generations. What you said about Master Zhāng Jièbīn's theory being wrong might not be appropriate. Master Zhāng was famous throughout the world; how could it have been easy for him to become so famous?!

I respond that true is true and false is false; this is the general rule of the world. Master Zhāng's contributions cannot be taken away, but there were aspects that did not follow the meaning of the Classic. Thus, I discuss it here to abolish what the ancient people hated. Why would I want to criticize unreasonably!?

或問，吾子數謂，背俞之寸方，古人不云適當，故紛紜之說起焉，吾子獨得經旨而知其適當歟，願聞其說焉。予應之曰：按皇莆氏王氏滑氏高武氏李氏馬氏皆曰，相去脊中為一寸五分，夫惟背之俞穴也者。醫之先務也，知其正路而不可不識其所在，故學者進步一差，秦胡遂隔絕。予是以辯明之爾。

---

at the level of Fèi Shù (UB 13), and the two lower corners would be on Xīn Shù (UB 15). Each time, the top of the triangle is moved down to the level of back transport point just found. For more on this, see the text of *Xíng Zhì Piān* (Plain Questions, Chapter 24) in appendix four on page 111.

Someone might ask: You frequently say that what ancient people[81] said about the cùn measurement of back transport points was inappropriate, and so a discrepancy arouse. You alone grasped the correct meaning of the Classic. I want to hear your theory.

I respond: Master Huángfǔ Mì, Master Wáng Bīng, Master Huá Bórén, Master Gāo Wǔ, Master Lǐ Chān, and Master Mǎ Shí all said that the back transport points were 1.5 cùn lateral to the spine.

The most urgent mission of a doctor is not just knowing the right way, but also its source. So if scholars miss one step, Qín and Hú will be separated.[82] Thus I want to clarify.[83]

---

81. Here the author is referring to his differences with doctors like Zhāng Jièbīn.
82. This means that things which should be considered at the same time are looked at separately. At the time of the Qín dynasty, the Hú was a specific minority group that fought with the Qín. Qín and Hú need to be looked at together, not as separate phenomenon. In this case, the two things that need to be considered together are the texts of *Bèi Shù Piān* and *Xíng Zhì Piān*. The difference of a half cùn in the distance of the inner bladder line from the spine may seem small but it makes a big difference clinically.
83. The author clarifies in the next chapter.

十五
Chapter 15

血氣形志篇讀草度之法者，"去半"之下加於"使之作四
方"，此五字而可視，便可知相柱之義也。柱字，彙腫與切
音，主掌也；掌，邪柱也。蓋兩邪柱相對，則上尖下廣，如
鱗形，似琴柱。故謂相柱也。有四方之物而斜，隅與隅等相
合，作三角之象，是謂相柱也。

Readers of the straw measurement method in *Xuè Qì Xíng Zhì Piān* have added
the words "making it into a square (*shǐ zhī zuò sì fāng* 使之作四方)" below
"remove half (*qù bàn* 去半)." From these five words, we can see the meaning of
"support each other." The word *zhù* 柱 (support) is pronounced with the zh of
zhǒng 腫 and the ù of *yù* 與[84]. It indicates *chèng* 掌. *Chèng* 掌 means *leaning to
supporting [each other]*.[85] When two things lean to support each other, the top is
sharp and the bottom is wide; this looks like a fish scale or the pillar[86] of a *qín*.[87]
Thus is the meaning of "supporting each other (*xiāng zhù* 相柱)."

A square shaped item folded diagonally so that corner and corner match each
other make the shape of a triangle. This is the meaning of *xiāng zhù* 相柱 (supporting each other).

---

84. Since Chinese is not a phonetic language, pronunciation was often given
using the opening consonant(s) of one familiar word and the final vowel(s) of
another familiar word. That is what is being done here.
85. This definition of *chèng* 掌 comes from *Guǎng Yùn • Qù Shēng • Yìng •
Chēng* 《廣韻·去聲·映·掌》.
86. This same character, *zhù* 柱, has many meanings. Pillar is one of the main
meanings. It also means, as we see here, the bridge or frets of a musical instrument like a *qín*. As a verb, it means to support, sustain, to bear or take the
weight of something.
87. A *qín* is a plucked seven-string Chinese musical instrument of zither family. The pillar of a *qín* has the same function as the bridge or frets of a guitar,
but it is triangular shaped. A *qín* has many of these pillars, one for each string.

經先度其兩乳間中折之，更以他草度，去半，使之作四方
已，即以兩隅相柱也。經文雖無干"使之作四方"之五字，
其意含蓄於去半已之中矣。是聖經之蘊奧也，未有四方之
物，而何合而得相柱歟？不然，則經文何指謂已，何以謂兩
隅，何合謂相柱乎哉！學者其察諸伏惟，雖恐憚於聖典，私
加"使之作四方"之五字於經文，而便於初學，不敢為達人
也。

The Classic says to first measure the distance between the nipples and fold [the straw] in the center. It alters another piece of straw, measuring, and half [of the length of straw] is removed. Next it makes a square, and once completed, it uses the two corners to support each other. Even though those five words "make it into a square (*shǐ zhī zuò sì fāng* 使之作四方)" do not exist in the text of the Classic, the meaning is contained in "once half is removed (*qù bàn yǐ* 去半 已)." This is the secret of the Classic; if there is no square-shaped item, how can it be matched to "support each other (*xiāng zhù* 相柱)"? Otherwise, what does this phrase indicate in the text of the Classic? Why does it say "two corners (*liǎng yú* 兩隅)" and "support each other (*xiāng zhù* 相柱)"? Even if scholars who perceived what was hidden felt intimidated [by making changes in] the sagely classics, they privately added "make it into a square (*shǐ zhī zuò sì fāng* 使 之作四方)" to benefit beginners, not daring to call themselves wise.

十六
Chapter 16

草度之方象國字解
The Images of [Anatomical] Measurement Methods Using Straw, Explained in Japanese[88]

愚按スルニ草度ノ法諸家紛紜ノ説多クシテ初學ヲ迷ハシム
唐ノ啓玄子王氷ヒトリ草度ノ法經旨ヲ得タリ以テ據トスベ
シ然レトモ其註文簡約ニシテ初學暁シカタシ

In my humble opinion, the [anatomical] measurement method using straw
is confusing. Schools offer different methods, and a beginner does not
know which one to choose. Wáng Bīng[89] of the *Táng* dynasty, also known as
Qǐxuánzǐ, was the one who developed the measuring system, and his method
is supposed to be the standard. However, his description was too simple for a
beginner to fully comprehend.

明ノ玄臺子馬註化ガ註證發微ニ草度ノ法解アリ其註文紛紜
トシテ正シカラズ惟ソノ云トコロ其兩隅當以三寸為闊則各
俞正合去脊一寸五分之度ト云フモノ背俞篇トアヘリ其他ノ
文言通シ難シ

Mǎ Shí[90] of the *Míng* dynasty, also known as Xuántáizǐ, wrote about the
measurement method in *Zhù Zhèng Fā Wēi*. His description is confusing and

---

88. The previous part of the book was written in literary Chinese, as educated
Japanese of the time were apt to do. But at this point, the author switches
to Japanese as he explains his own methods in more detail. There is some
repetition here, but it is written in Japanese, not Chinese. The author probably
wanted to be sure his students understood.
89. Wáng Bīng edited *Sù Wèn* and put it more or less in the form we have
received today. His *hào*-name was Qǐxuánzǐ.
90. Mǎ Shí 馬蒔 wrote *Sù Wèn Zhù Zhèng Fā Wēi*《素問注證發微》. His
hào-name was Xuántáizǐ.

incorrect. For example, he wrote "when the two corners are 3 cùn apart, the measurement of each transport point is exactly 1.5 cùn away from the spine."[91] The other sentences are hard to comprehend as well.

同世張介賓類經ノ大事ヲ成セリ然シテ草度ノ法解アレトモ
其法象ヲ錯リ背俞ノ寸法ヲ誤マル百有餘年誤リヲ世ニ傳ル
トイヘトモ敢テ其非ヲ正ス者有ルコトヲ聞カズ嘆スベキカ
ナ今予獨リ其非ヲ正サント欲ス故ニ初學童蒙ノタメニ和語
ヲ以テ草度ノ法ヲ圖解スルコト左ノ如シ

Zhāng Jièbīn of the same era wrote a large collection called *Lèi Jīng*. In the collection, the measuring method is described. Unfortunately, the images that depict the method are mistaken, and the measurement of back transport points is incorrect. Although the mistake has been in the public for over a hundred years, I don't know of anybody who has tried to correct it. This is the reason I felt obligated to correct the measurement mistake and explain the measurement method in the Japanese language so that young students understand it.

血氣形志篇曰欲知背俞先度其両乳間中折之更以他草度去半
已即以両隅相柱也云云

Sù Wèn, Chapter 24 (*Xíng Zhì Piān*, Blood, Qi, Body, and Spirit) states, "If one wants to know [the location of] the back transport points, first measure [the distance between] the nipples [with a piece of straw] and fold it in the center. Alter another piece of straw, measuring [it to the same length], and once half [the length of straw] is removed, use the two corners to support each other," etc.

先度其両乳間トハ度ハ量ナリ古ヘハ細長草ヲ以テ量リシナ
リ今ハ細長キ紙ヲ用ユ便利ナル故ナレバナリ紙ヲ細ク截ツ
テ先ズ両乳ノアイダヲ量ル是ヲ八寸トス

---

91. There are some differences between this and what Mǎ Shí actually wrote: 其兩隅當以三寸為闊則各俞正合去脊一寸五分之度. The Japanese author, Cūnshàng Qīnfāng Zōngzhàn, had: 其兩隅當以三寸為闊則各俞正合去脊一寸五分之度. (The differences are underlined.) One reason the author may have found it confusing is that these characters were different.

In the phrase "first measure [the distance between] the nipples," the character *dù* 度 is a synonym for *liàng* 量, which means to measure. In the old days, a thin piece of straw was used. Nowadays, thin strips of paper should suffice for convenience. Cut a thin strip of paper and measure the distance between the nipples. The distance is 8 cùn.

中折之トハ右ノ乳ノ間ヲ量リシ八寸ノ紙ヲ真中カヨリ二ツ
ニ折レバカタカタ四寸トナル也

"Fold it in the center" means to take the 8 cùn strip of paper which was used to measure the distance between the nipples in the paragraph above and fold it in two at the exact center. The distance is 4 cùn.

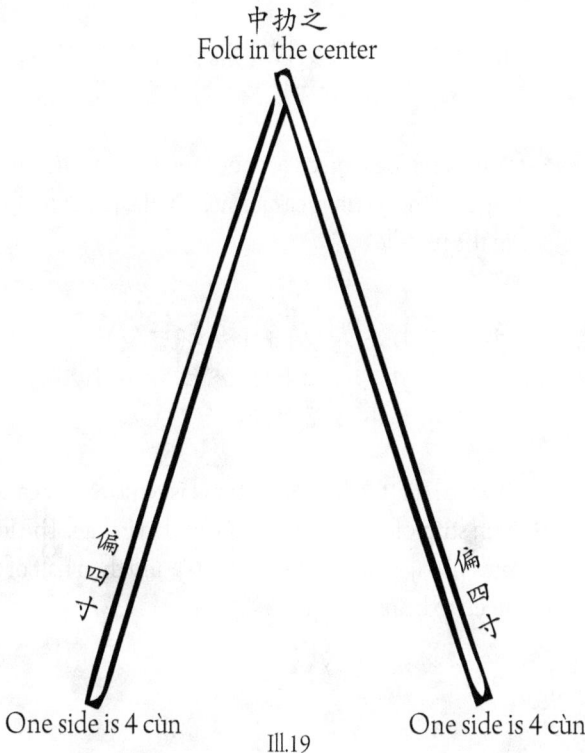

中折之
Fold in the center

偏四寸

偏四寸

One side is 4 cùn

One side is 4 cùn

Ill.19

八寸ノ細紙ヲ二ツニヲレバカタカタ四寸ツツニナルナリ圖
上ノコトシ

When an 8 cùn long thin strip of paper is folded in two, each side becomes 4 cùn long, as shown in the diagram above.

更以他草度トハ更ハ改ナリ他ハ別ナリ改メテ別ニ外ノ細キ
紙ヲ以テ前ノ中ニ折ル四寸ノ紙ニクラベ是ヲモ又四寸トス
圖左ノ如シ

In the phrase "Alter another piece of straw, measuring," 更 (change, replace, more) really should be 改 (alter, change, improve). 他 (other, another) should be 別 (different, separate). You need to take a separate thin strip of paper and measure 4 cùn, using the 4 cùn long strip of paper that was previously created by folding [the 8 cùn strip] in two, as shown below.

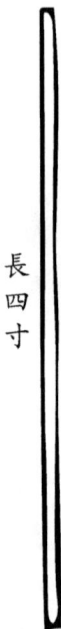

更ラニ別ノ紙ヲ以テ前ノカタカタ四寸ニクラ
ベハカリ取ルナリ

Alter a separate piece of paper and measure 4 cùn by comparing it to the 4 cùn measurement of the paper that was folded in the middle.

去半已トハ右ノ四寸ノ紙ヲ又マン中ヨリ二ツ
ニヲル也二ツニ折レバニ寸トナルカタカタ捨
テニ寸ヲトル故ニ半バヲ去ルト云

"Once half [the length of straw] is removed" means that the 4 cùn strip of paper needs to be folded in half. The folding creates [two] 2 cùn long [segments], and then half of the paper need to be removed.

長
四
寸

Four cùn long

Ill.20

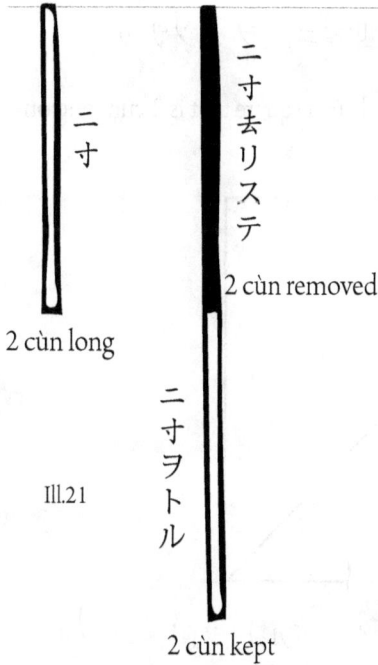

二寸

2 cùn long

Ill.21

二寸去リステ

2 cùn removed

二寸ヲトル

2 cùn kept

上ミ二寸ヲ切リステ下モ二寸ヲ用ユ

Cut off the upper 2 cùn and remove it; keep the lower 2 cùn.

此ノ二寸ノ紙ヲ以テ法トシ紙ヲ四角ニ切テ二寸四方トナス是ヲスヂカヒニ折リ角ト角トカサ子合セテ三角ウロコノ象トナスナリ即チ以両隅相柱也トハ是ヲ云フナリ隅ハ角ナリ四角ノ紙ヲ角ト角トヲアハスレハ三角トナル此ノ三角トナリタル形ヲ柱スト云フナリ圖左ノ如シ.

Using this 2 cùn long strip of paper as the guide, cut [another piece of] paper into a square that is 2 cùn long on all four sides. Fold this paper diagonally to make the corners line up. This should make a triangle that is shaped like a fish scale. In the text "use the two corners to support each other," 隅 means corners, and 柱 (support) indicates that corners support each other to form a triangle from the square. A diagram is shown below.

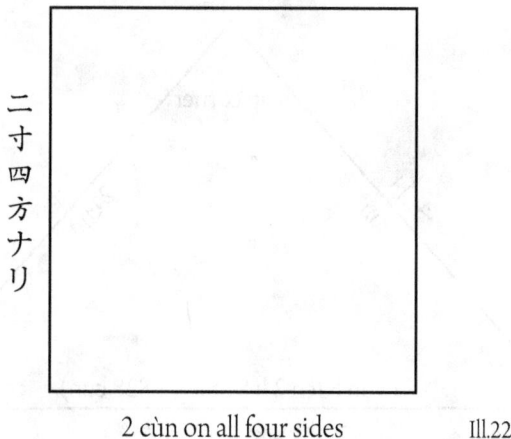

二寸四方ナリ

2 cùn on all four sides

Ill.22

79

右ノ二寸ノ紙ヲ法トシ如此二寸四方ニ紙ヲタツナリ

Use the 2 cùn strip of paper as the guide and cut a square that is 2 cùn long on all four sides.

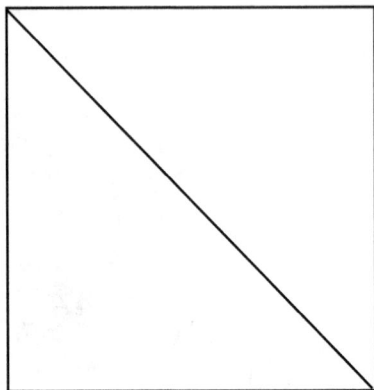

Ill.23

二寸四方ノ紙ヲ圖ノ如クスヂカイニ折ル是ヲ斜メニ折ルト云フ也是上ミニ云フトコロノ角ト角トアハスルナリ

Fold the 2 cùn square paper diagonally. As stated in the phrase, "the corners support each other."

三隅之象
Image of the three corners

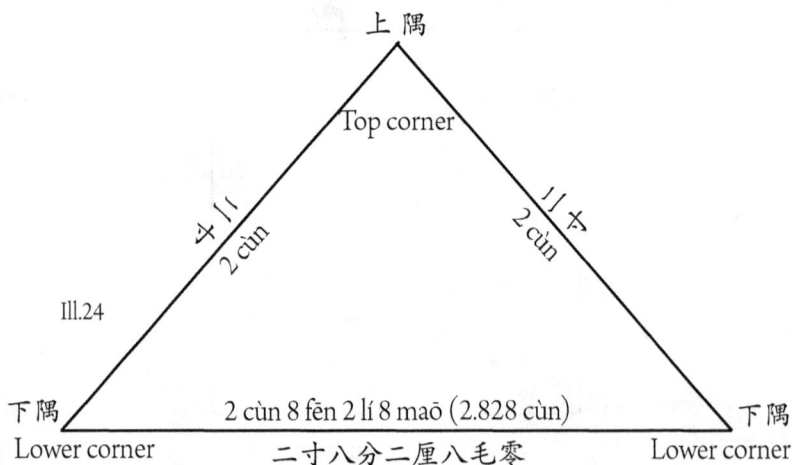

上 隅
Top corner

4 厘
2 cùn

2 cùn
4 厘

Ill.24

下 隅
Lower corner

下 隅
Lower corner

2 cùn 8 fēn 2 lí 8 maō (2.828 cùn)
二寸八分二厘八毛零

80

隅ハ角ナリ三隅ハ三角ナリ上ミノスヂカイニ折リタル如此
三角ニ成リ鱗形ノ如ク琴柱ニ似タリ經文ノ柱ノ字ハ是ノ義
ナリ

隅 (corner) means angle. Therefore, "three corners" is a triangle that is formed
from folding the paper diagonally. It is shaped like a fish scale, and it also resembles a bridge for a *koto* (琴柱). The character, 柱 (support, pillar) indicates a
bridge for a *koto* [*qín* in Chinese] in the text of the Classic.

乃擧以度其背令其一隅居上齊脊大推両隅在下當其下隅者肺
之俞也云云

"Then hold the measuring [straw] on the back. Make the upper corner even
with Dà Zhuī (Dū 14) on the spine. The two lower corners will be at the back
transport point of the lungs (UB 13)," etc.[92]

右ノ三隅ノ象ヲアケテ以テ背ヲ
ハカル上ミノ尖リヲ大推ニアテ
下モ両傍ノトカリ便チ背ノ二行
ニアタルナリ圖ノ如シ

When you measure the back, hold the triangle and align the top with Dà Zhuī (Dū
14). The bottom two angles should touch
the two channels as shown here:

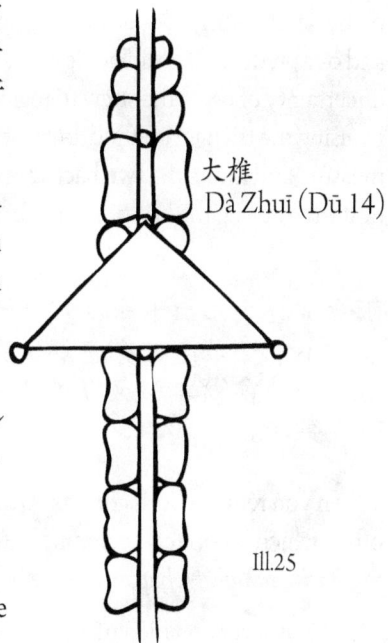

大椎
Dà Zhuī (Dū 14)

Ill.25

下両隅ノ端シニ点ス両俞相去ル
コト全ク三寸ナリ是レ背俞篇ト
相合ス

The two angles at the bottom are at the
location of both transport points. They are

---

92. This is a continuation of *Sù Wèn*, Chapter 24 (*Xíng Zhì Piān*, Blood, Qi,
Body, and Spirit).

3 cùn apart, just as described in the *Back Transport Chapter* (*Líng Shū* Chapter 51).

復下一度心之俞也云云

"Repeat one time below for the back transport point of the heart (UB 15)," etc.[93]

是レ背俞篇トアハズ按ズルニ心之俞也以下ノ經文ウタガウハ缺語アラン背俞篇トアハズ先輩ノ註解モ詳カナラズ予ココ以テ疑ヒヲ缺テタタ草度三隅ノ象ヲ用テ復下一度復下一度ノ法ヲ用ヒズ三隅象下ノ両隅ヲ用テ背俞ノ二行ヲ量リテ其両隅ノハシニ点ス

This statement does not match what it says in the *Back Transport Chapter*. I suspect that some text is missing after "心之俞也 the back transport point of the heart (UB 15)." It does not follow what the *Back Transport Chapter* says, and our predecessors did not leave us a detailed explanation. I disregard that uncertainty of using the straw triangle measurement to "repeat one time below." By using the triangle method, but not the repeat-one-time-below method, I measure and locate the two back transport lines. I mark the two corners on the bottom by using the bottom two corners of the triangle.

兩俞アヒ去ルコト全ク三寸ナリ背俞篇トアヘリ故ニ背俞篇ヲ主トシテ草度モ亦三隅ノ象下ノ両隅ヲ用ルナリ五藏俞ニ点セハ背俞篇ニシタガイ某ノ俞ハ某ノ推下ニアリ幾度モ脊推ヲ数エ正ク詳ニシテ誤ルコト勿レ

When you remove both corners,[94] [the marks] are 3 cùn [away from each other, which is correct] according to the *Back Transport Chapter*. As written in the *Back Transport Chapter*, use the bottom two corners of the triangle. When

---

93. This is a continuation of *Sù Wèn*, Chapter 24 (*Xíng Zhì Piān*, Blood, Qi, Body, and Spirit).
94. The text says "When you remove both transport-points (兩俞)..." which must be an error for "When you remove both corners (兩隅)..."

you locate [the transport-points of] the five *zàng*-organs, know that the five *zàng*-organ transport-points are at the level of the lower [border] of a vertebra. Count the vertebrae correctly and precisely to avoid mistakes.

譬ヘハ肝俞ニ点セハ九推ノ下脊中ニ假点シテカノ三隅ノ象
ヲ以テ堅テニニツニ折リ下両隅ヲ合セ

如此折メノ下角ヲ假点ニ合
セ左右ニヒラキ両隅ノ端シ
ニ点ス両点相去ルコト全ノ
三寸ナリ二行通シテ皆是ニ
倣エ是レ予ガ臆説ニ非ス背
俞形志ノ二篇並行シ相悖ラ
ザルナリ

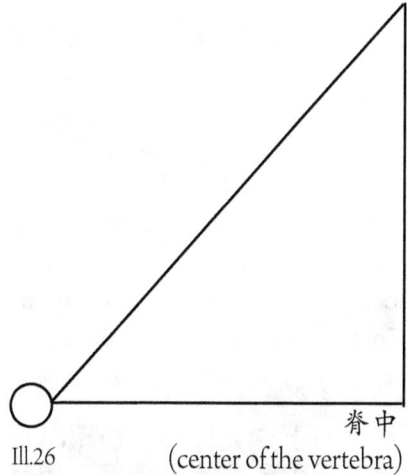

Ill.26

脊中
(center of the vertebra)

For example, to mark the liver transport-point (UB 18), make a temporary mark under the ninth vertebra. Fold the triangle tightly in half so that the bottom corners meet. Align the bottom corner of the fold to the temporary mark and open up the triangle. Mark the edges of the two angles and then remove the triangle. The distance is 3 cùn. The lines of both [sides of the channel] are determined based on this. This is how I know that this theory is not just a popular assumption. *Back Transport Chapter* (*Líng Shū*, Chapter 51) and *Body and Spirit Chapter* (*Sù Wèn*, Chapter 24) concur and do not disagree.

又一法アリ胸腹背ニ鍼灸ヲ施ス横ニ開ク骨度ノ寸法ハ某ノ
両乳ノ間ヲ細紙ヲ以テ量リ八寸トス四ツニ折リ一折ヲ去ル
三折ヲ取リマンナカヨリ二ツニ折ル偏々三寸ナリ折メヲ脊
中ニアテ左右ニ開キ其ハシヲ背ノ三行トヲリトス

There is another method. When you perform acupuncture and moxibustion on the chest, abdomen, and back, you may measure the bones in the following fashion. Measure between the nipples with a thin strip of paper and call it 8 cùn. Fold the paper in quarters, remove one quarter, and leave three quarters. Fold the remaining [three-quarters piece, which would be 6 cùn] in half to create 3 cùn. Align the center fold with the spine, open the paper, and at the end of the paper, mark the third line [the outer urinary bladder line] on the back.

譬ハ魄戸ニ点セハ三推ノ脊中ニ假点シ彼ノ細紙ノ折メヲ假
点ニアテ左右ニ開キ其端ニ点ス三行通リ各俞皆コレニ倣エ
三行ハ上附分ヨリ下秩邊ニ至リ各脊中ヲ相去ルコト三寸ナ
リ

For example, in order to mark Pò Hù (UB 42), place a temporary mark in the center at the third vertebra. Align the fold of the thin strip of paper with the temporary mark, open the paper to the right and left, and mark on the two points at the edges. These mark the third line. Each transport-point should be located in the same fashion. The third line extends from Fù Fēng (UB 41) to Zhì Biān (UB 54), and the points are 3 cùn from the center of the spine.

二行ハ上ミ大杼ヨリ白環ニ至リ脊中ヲ相去コト各一寸五分
ナリ皆両乳八寸ノ骨度ヲ用ユ二行三行ニ点セハ背俞篇説ク
所ノ如ク肺俞ハ三焦ノ間ニアリト云ハ三推ノ下四推ノ上脊
中ニ假リ点シ点ヨリ横ニ開クコト一寸五分ナリ肺俞以下コ
レニ倣エ脊推ヲ数ルコト再三詳ニシテ差フコト勿レ

The second line starts from Dà Zhù (UB 11) and reaches Bái Huán (UB 30). This line is 1.5 cùn from the center of the spine. Each point is located using the measurement method obtained from the 8 cùn distance between the nipples. As you mark the second and third lines, you see the lung transport-point (UB 13) is located in the space of the third vertebra[95] as the *Back Transport Chapter* indicates. A temporary mark should be placed between the third and fourth vertebra, then open [the strip of paper] horizontally to 1.5 cùn away from the spine; this is the lung transport-point (UB 13). The rest should be located the same way. Make sure to count the vertebrae repeatedly to avoid mistakes.

---

95. The text has *sān jiāo* 三焦 (triple burner), which must be a typographical error for *sān zhuī* 三椎 (third vertebra).

十七

Chapter Seventeen

脊骨二十一節アリ大推ヨリ尾骶骨ニ至リ長コト三尺ナリ上
ミ七節中七節下七節長短同シカラズ中七節ハ推節ナガシ上
七節ハ中ヨリ短ク下七節ハ又短シ按スルニ甲乙經註證發微
類經等ニ脊節ノ長短ヲ説クコト詳ナリ

There are twenty-one spinous processes on the vertebral column. The distance
is 3 chǐ from Dà Zhuī (Dū 14) to the coccyx. The upper seven, middle seven,
and lower seven are different in size. The middle seven are longer. The upper
seven are shorter than the middle ones, and the lower seven are even shorter.
I recall that there are detailed descriptions of the vertebral length in *Jiǎ Yǐ Jīng*,
Zhù Zhèng Fā Wēi, and *Lèi Jīng*.

類經ニ曰上節各長一寸四分分ノ一即チ一寸四分一釐ナリ共
九寸八分七釐中七節各長一寸六分一厘共一尺一寸二分七厘
第十四節與臍平也下七節各長一寸二分六釐共八寸八分二厘
總共二尺九寸九分六釐不足四厘者有零未盡云愚按スルニ脊
推尤モ数エガタシ三子ノ説尤モ是ナリ然トモ初學ハ其眞ニ
當リガタシ予コレヲ師ニ得タリ

According to *Lèi Jīng*, the distance between the upper processes is 1.4 cùn
and one tenth, which is 1.41 cùn. The total length [of all seven] is 9.87 cùn.
The distance between the middle seven processes is 1.61 cùn, and the total
length is 11.27 cùn. The fourteenth process $[L_2]$ is at the level of the umbilicus. The distance between the lower seven processes is 1.26 cùn, totaling 8.82
cùn. The total length of all of them is 29.96 cùn. This is missing four lí [which
would bring the total to 30 cùn] due to uncounted small fractions. I think that
vertebrae are difficult to count. The three scholars[96] mention this as well in their

---

96. This probably refers to Wáng Bīng, Mǎ Shí, and Zhāng Jièbīn, who were
all mentioned in Chapter 16.

books. A beginner really has hard time with counting vertebrae. I learned it from my teacher.

別ニ口授アリ

There are additional oral instructions [not given here].

十八
Chapter Eighteen

或人問テ曰吾子カ云フトコロノ草度ノ法二寸ヲ以テ法トシ
四角作リ二寸四方トシ是ヲ斜メニ折角ト角ト合セテ三隅ノ
象トナスト云コト經文ニ見エズ證トスベキナシ恐クハ臆説
ナラン予答テ曰經文ノ蘊奥容易ニ暁スベカラズ篤ク學ヒ深
ク思ヒ久フシテ然後ニ意味ノ深長ヲ覚ベシ

Someone asked me "According to your measurement method with straw, you establish 2 cùn as the guide and create a square that is 2 cùn on each side. Then, you fold it diagonally, align the angles, and make a triangular shape. This procedure is not found in the text, and there is no proof that this is correct. Is this just an assumption?" I answered, "The profound nature of the text cannot be easily understood. After you study it sincerely and ponder it deeply for a while, the deep meaning becomes clear to you."

去半已即以両隅相柱ストキハ柱セザル前去半是ヲ法トシ四
方ニ作リ已リ両隅ヲ以テ相柱スベシ柱スルトキハ三隅ノ象
トナル蓋シ三隅ノ象ハ四隅ヨリ生ス四角ナルモノ角ト角ト
ヲ合テ三角生ス是レ四隅文中ニ含蓄ス古文辞ノ語意カクノ
如シ學者熟讀玩味シテ後得ベシ

The phrase "once half [the length of straw] is removed, use the two corners to support each other" conveys the idea of removing half [the length of the straw] before [using the corners] to support each other. You should use the half [of the length] as a guide to create a square. Then, you place two corners [of the square] on each other. When "supporting each other," a triangle is created from a square. The fact that a triangle is created from a square by placing one corner on another corner is implied in the sentence. Ancient Chinese texts often imply things like this, and a scholar must read them carefully and ponder for a while in order to understand the full meaning.

柱ノ字字彙ニ本音直呂切音除上声楹也家ノ柱ラナリ又腫與
切音主掌也掌ハ邪柱ナリ邪ノ字ナナメト訓ス邪柱ハハシラ
ノ斜ニユガミタルナリ經文ノ相柱ストハ相ハアヒ對スル義
ナリ二本ノ邪柱アヒ對スレバ上ミ尖リ下ヒロシ鱗ノナリノ
如ク琴ノ柱ニ似タリ故ニ柱云

The character 柱 is pronounced *zhǔ* besides the above pronunciation according to a dictionary. It is synonymous with *yíng* 楹, which is the pillar of a house. Also, when pronounced *zhù*, it is the same as the character *chēng* 掌, which means to support or to prop up.[97] The components of a compound phrase are 邪 and 柱. *Xié* 邪 can be read as *naname*, which means "*xié* 斜 slanting." The phrase, 邪柱 is therefore a slanting pillar. In the text, the phrase 相 (each other) 柱 (meaning both *pillar* and *support*) means two slanting pillars supporting each other. This formation tapers to a point on top and opens wide at the bottom. It is shaped like a fish scale and resembles a bridge for a *koto*.

---

97. In Chinese, sometimes the same character has different pronunciations associated with different meanings. Here, 柱 is pronounced *zhǔ* (third tone) or *zhù* (fourth tone). The author's dictionary does not agree with Paul W. Kroll's *Dictionary of Classical and Medieval Chinese* (Brill, 2015). On page 619, it states that *zhǔ* means to support, sustain, or bear the weight of something while *zhù* denotes a pillar, post, or column of a building, or the bridge of a musical instrument. The author can perhaps be forgiven as Chinese is not his native language. Neither does this take away from his point that 柱 carries both meanings.

十九
Chapter Nineteen

張介賓考ル草度三隅ノ象經旨ニ彷彿タリトイヘトモ其象竪
長ク横廣シ圖左ノ如シ

Zhāng Jièbīn's version of the triangular shape follows the context of the book, but it seems longer vertically and wider horizontally as shown in the following figure.

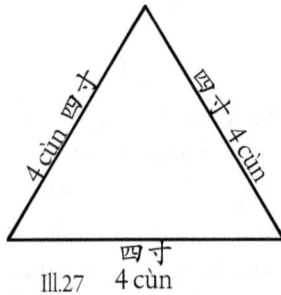

Ill.27　四寸　4 cùn

八寸中折ノ長草ヲタテニ立テ四寸ノ短草ヲ下ニヲキ中折ノ
両端ニ加エテ三角ノ象トナス此ノ圖ヲ以テ背ノ俞穴ヲ量ル
トキハ穴處ノビテ各々其本位ニアタラズ背俞篇トアハズ用
ヒガタシ

The 8 cùn longer straw is folded in the middle. It is placed vertically on top of a 4 cùn shorter straw. By placing the two ends of the folded straw on the ends of the short straw, a triangle is formed. When you try to measure back transport-points with this configuration, it is too far away from the points. It does not hit any of the back transport-points and does not match the description in the *Back Transport Chapter*.

予ガ考ル草度三隅ノ象下ノ両隅相去コト三寸背俞篇ニ合ス
ト云エドモタテテ短クシテ肺俞以下復タ一度ヲ下スノ法ニア
ハズ彼ニ因テ是ヲ見レハ草度ノ法疑ヒアリテ用ヒガタシ斯

88

以ソノ疑ヲ闕ヒテ用ヒズ背俞篇疑ナキヲ以テ正キ據トシテ
二行背中ヨリ一寸五分三行脊中ヨリ三寸トスルナリ是レ經
ノ本旨ナリ疑フコト勿レ蓋シ俞穴ヲ取ルニ某ノ俞ハ某推下
ノ左右ニアリ能推節ヲ数エ正シ取ルベシ推節数エ難シ口授
アリ

My version of the measuring method with straw is 3 cùn wide between the
bottom two corners. It agrees with what the *Back Transport Chapter* says, but
the height of the triangle is too short to repeat the process to locate the back
transport-points below the lung transport-point (UB 13). This does not mean
that the *Back Transport Chapter* is incorrect. Without a doubt, the second line
[on the back, the inner bladder line] is 1.5 cùn from the spine, and the third line
[on the back, the outer bladder line] is 3 cùn from the spine. You must remem-
ber that transport-points are located bilaterally under the vertebrae. Vertebrae
must be counted correctly, but counting vertebrae correctly is difficult.

口授アリ

There is oral instruction [not given here].

二十

Chapter Twenty

再按草度ノ法介賓經旨ヲ觀ルコト錯レリ故ニ草度ノ法象四
寸三面ノ形象トナル是ヲ以テ五藏ノ俞穴ヲ量ル両穴相ヒ去
ルコト四寸ナリ尚又四寸トナスベキノ証トシテ背俞篇ニ所
謂皆俠脊相去三寸所ト云フヲ據トシテ圖翼曰云云前ニ見エ
タリ

As I revisited Zhāng Jièbīn's work, I found that he mistakenly created an equilateral triangle that is 4 cùn on each side. When you use this triangle to measure the location of the transport-points of the five *zàng*-organs, the distance
between two back transport-points ends up being 4 cùn. As the proof that the
distance should be 4 cùn, Zhāng used a phrase from the *Back Transport Chapter*,
"each is 3 cùn from the spine." I have seen this in *Lèi Jīng Tú Yì*.

其俠脊ト云經文ニ因テ脊骨一寸除脊外ヨリ量ル者經旨ニ非
ス自見臆説ナリ予經文中ヲ閲ルニ俠ノ字ヲ加フコト背俞篇
ノミニ非ス氣府論足ノ陽明曰俠鳩尾外云云俠胃脘云云俠臍
云云下臍二寸俠之云云此俠也是ヲノゾカバ何ン寸トシテ除
クベキヤ介賓コレヲ如何學者コレヲ思ヘ脊骨ハ中ニ在リ二
行三行両旁ヲメクル鳩尾胃脘臍トモニ中ニ在リ胃經ソノ両
旁ヲメクル故ニ俠ト云フナリ俠ノ字深意ナシ介賓ガ説恐ラ
クハ經旨ニアラズ故ニ予脊骨ヲノゾカズ脊中ヨリハカル者
此レガタメナリ

Zhāng assumed that in the text of the Classic, "俠脊 (to clasp or pinch the
spine)" suggests omitting 1 cùn as the width of a vertebra and measuring from
the outside of a vertebra. However, this is not the case, in my opinion. I see this
character, *jiā* 俠 (to clasp or pinch), used frequently throughout the text of the
Back Transport Chapter. For instance, in the leg yángmíng section of *Discussion of Qì Mansions* (*Sù Wèn*, Chapter 59), *jiā* 俠 (to clasp or pinch) is found
in phrases like "pinching lateral to Jiū Wěi (Rèn 15)," "pinching Wèi Wǎn [an

alternative name for Rèn 12 or Rèn 13])," "pinching the umbilicus," and 2 cùn under the umbilicus and pinching it. The character *jiā* 俠 does not indicate omitting any cùn from the measurement. How could a scholar like Zhāng Jiébīn think like that!? Just like the spine is located in the center with two channels lateral to it, the stomach channel is located on both sides lateral to Jiū Wěi (Rèn 15), Wèi Wǎn [an alternative name for Rèn 12 or Rèn 13], and the umbilicus. *Jiā* 俠 merely indicates "existing on both sides." This character does not have any deeper meaning. I disregard Zhāng Jiébīn's theory and think that the measurement should be from the center of the spine. These are my thoughts.

The end of *Kotsu Do Sei Go Zu Setsu*

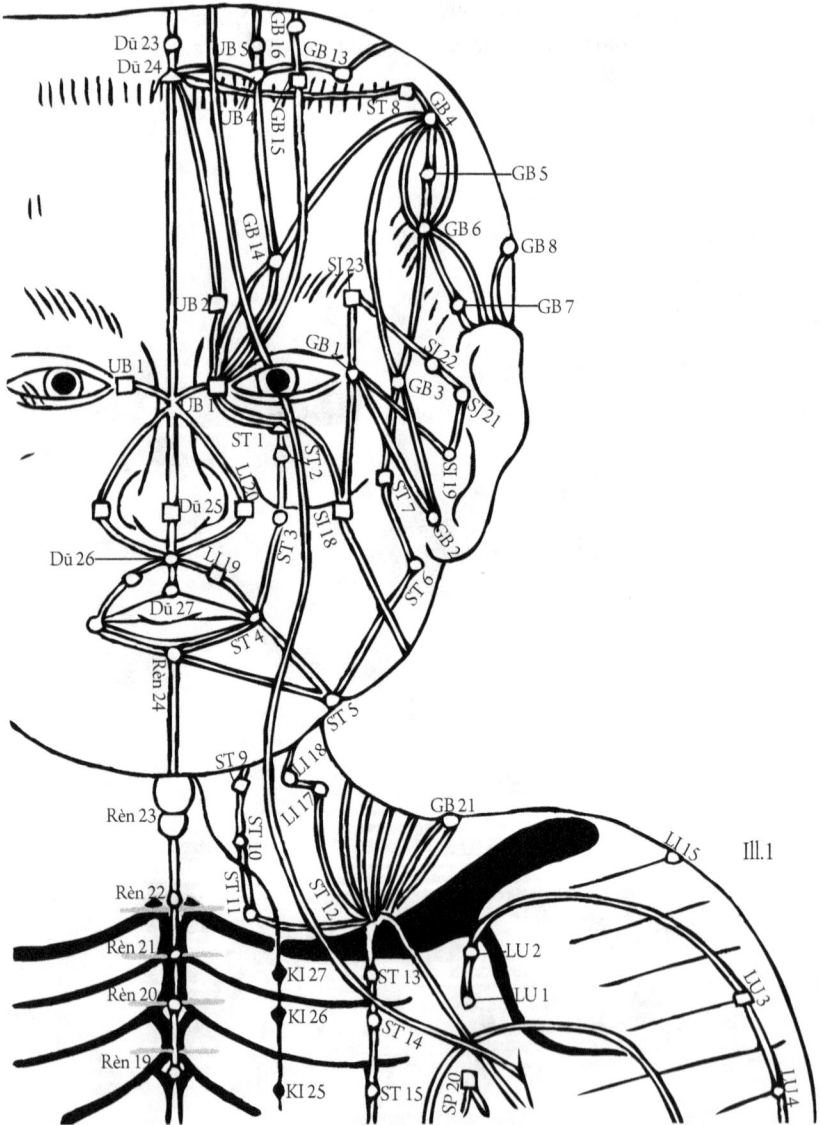

Ill. 1

92

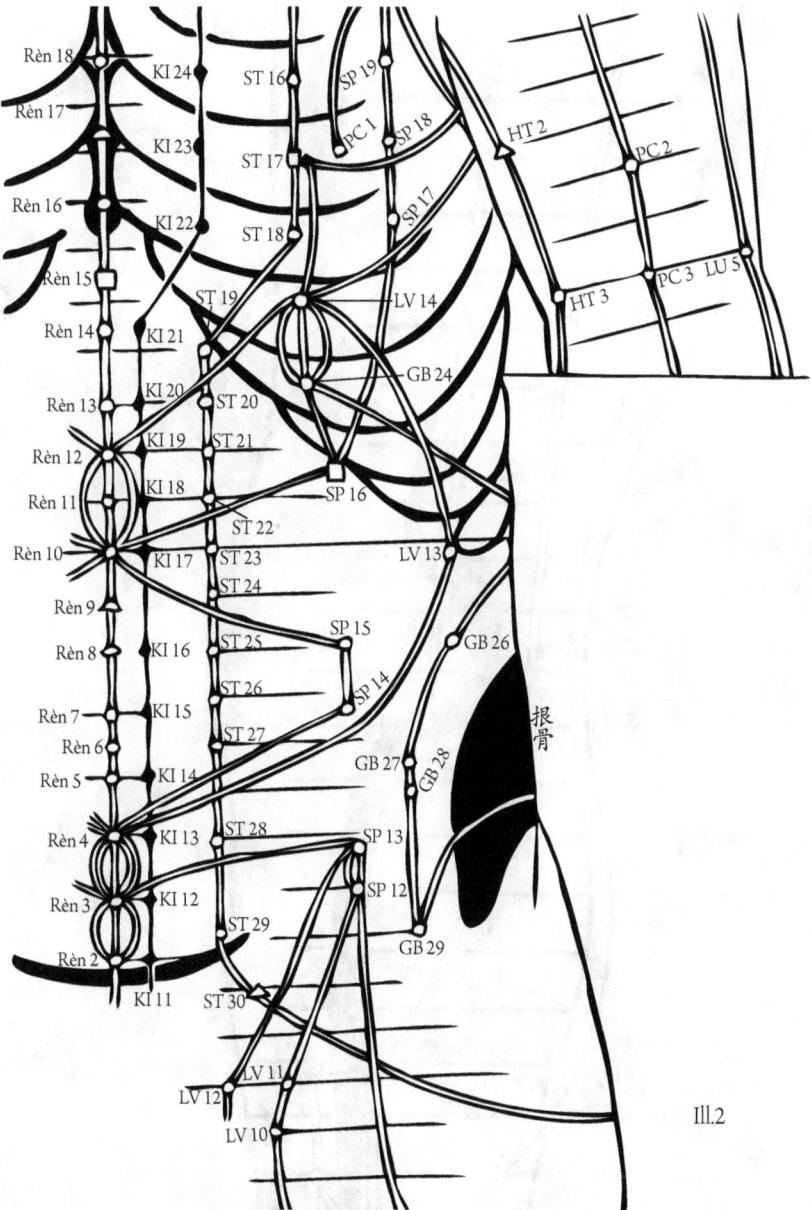

Rèn 18
KI 24
ST 16
SP 19
Rèn 17
PC 1
SP 18
HT 2
PC 2
KI 23
ST 17
Rèn 16
KI 22
ST 18
SP 17
Rèn 15
ST 19
LV 14
HT 3
PC 3 LU 5
Rèn 14
KI 21
Rèn 13
KI 20
ST 20
GB 24
Rèn 12
KI 19
ST 21
Rèn 11
KI 18
SP 16
ST 22
Rèn 10
KI 17
ST 23
LV 13
ST 24
Rèn 9
Rèn 8
KI 16
ST 25
SP 15
GB 26
ST 26
SP 14
Rèn 7
KI 15
ST 27
Rèn 6
GB 27
GB 28
Rèn 5
KI 14
根骨
Rèn 4
KI 13
ST 28
SP 13
Rèn 3
KI 12
SP 12
ST 29
GB 29
Rèn 2
KI 11
ST 30
LV 11
LV 12
LV 10

Ill.2

93

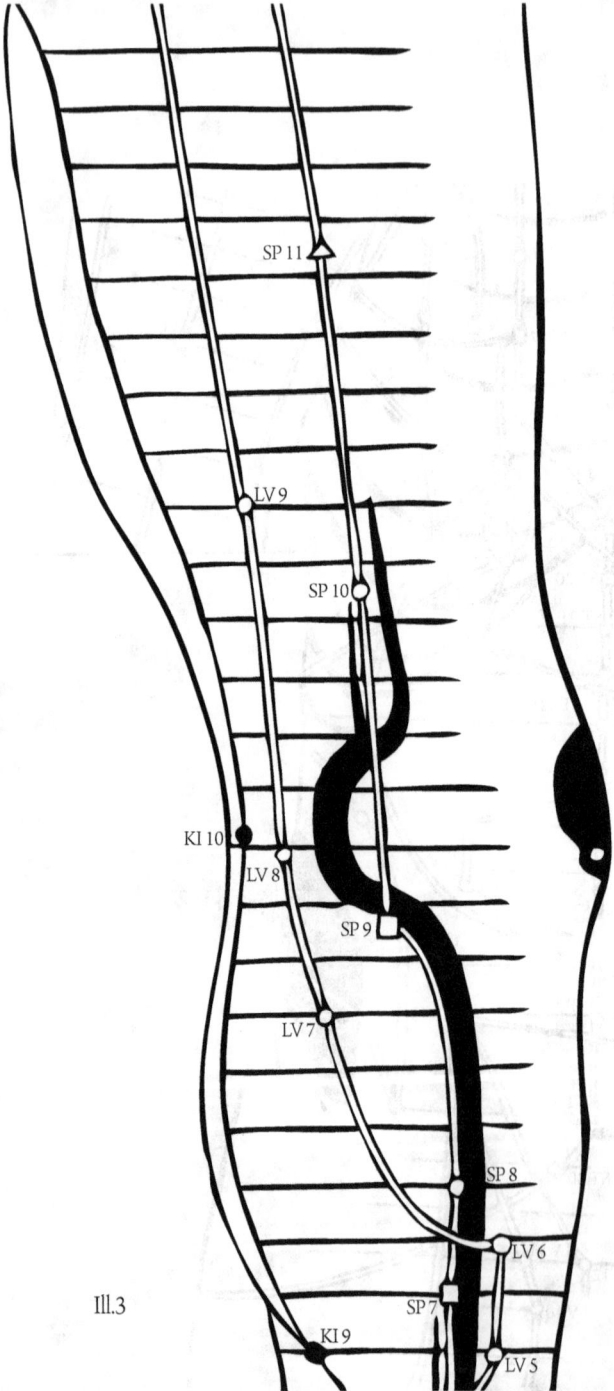

Ill.3

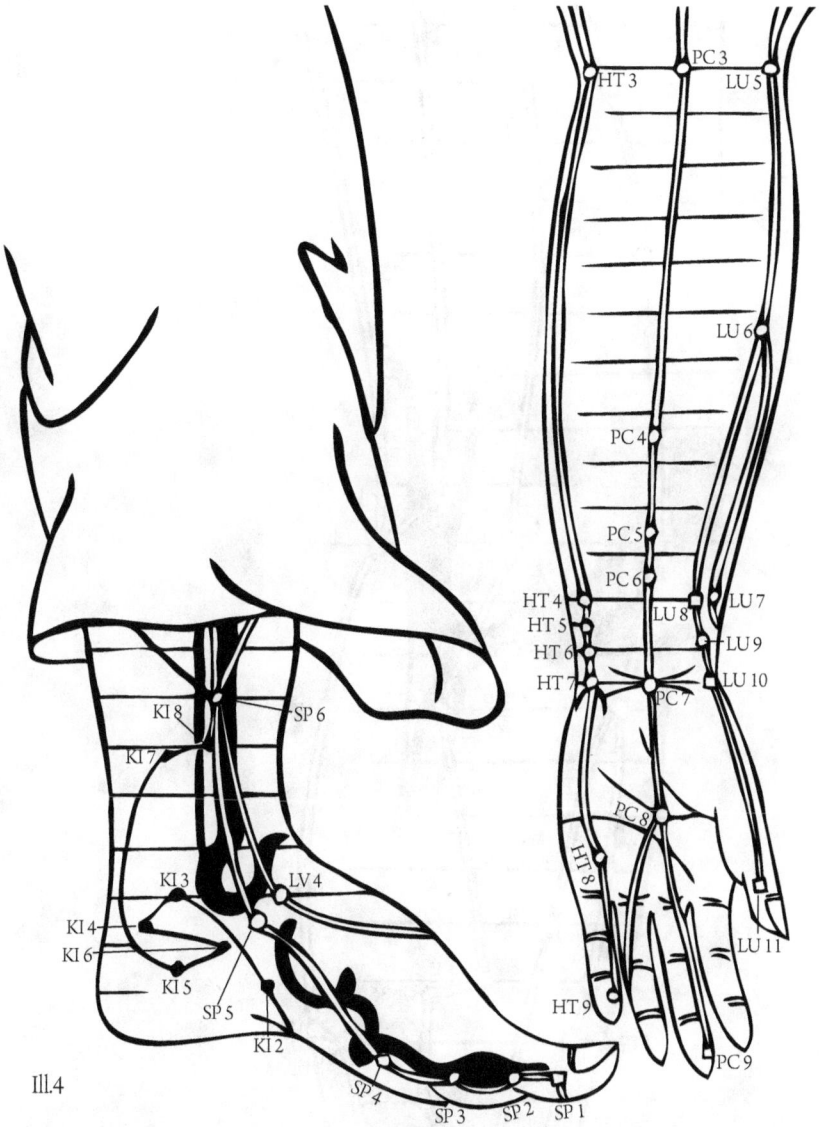

Ill.4

95

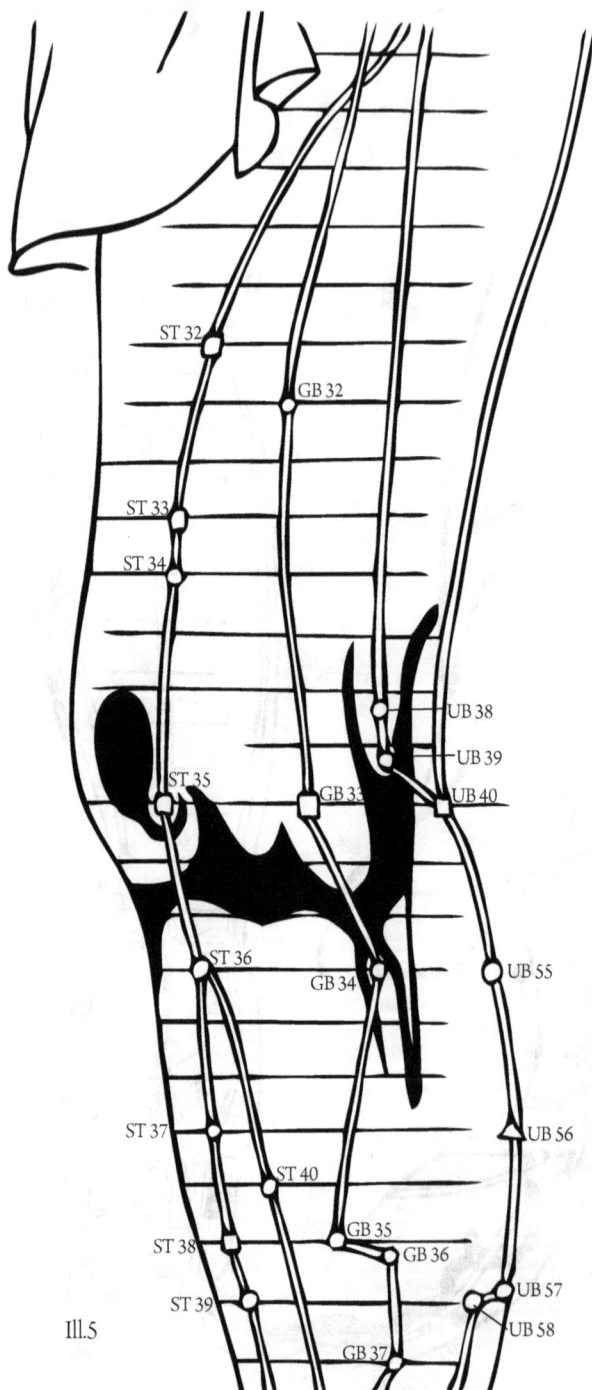

Ill.5

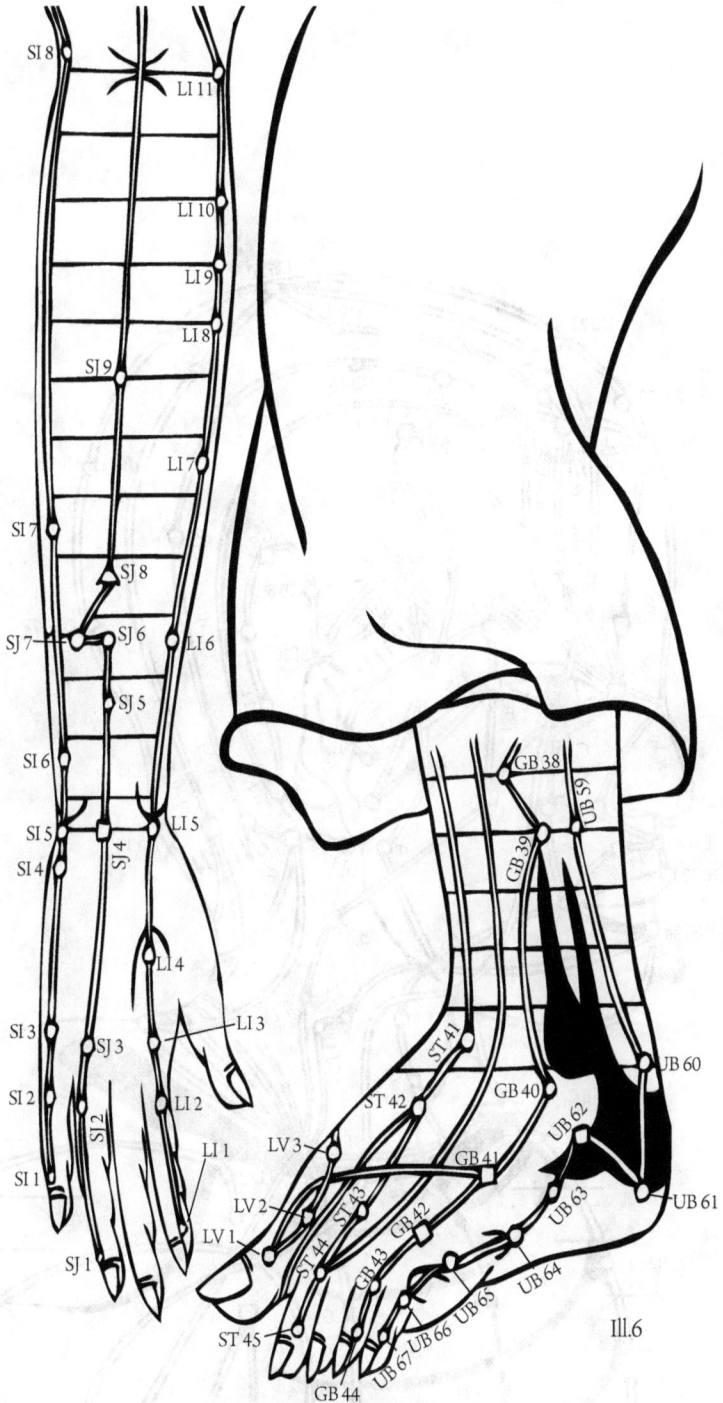

SI 8
LI 11
LI 10
LI 9
LI 8
SJ 9
LI 7
SI 7
SJ 8
SJ 7
SJ 6
LI 6
SJ 5
SI 6
SI 5
SJ 4
LI 5
SI 4
LI 4
SI 3
SJ 3
LI 3
SI 2
SJ 2
LI 2
SI 1
LI 1
SJ 1

GB 38
UB 59
GB 39
ST 41
UB 60
ST 42
GB 40
UB 62
LV 3
GB 41
UB 63
LV 2
ST 43
UB 61
LV 1
ST 44
GB 42
UB 64
GB 43
UB 65
ST 45
UB 67
UB 66
GB 44

Ill.6

97

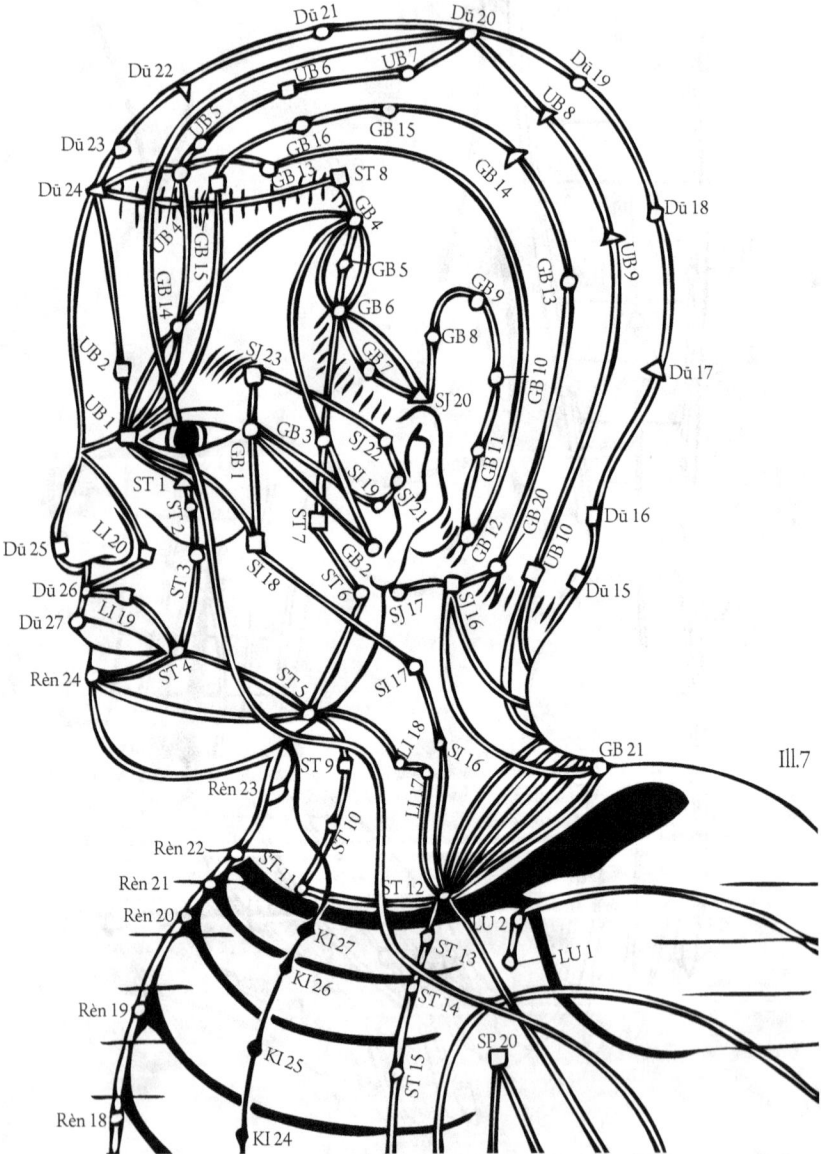

Ill.7

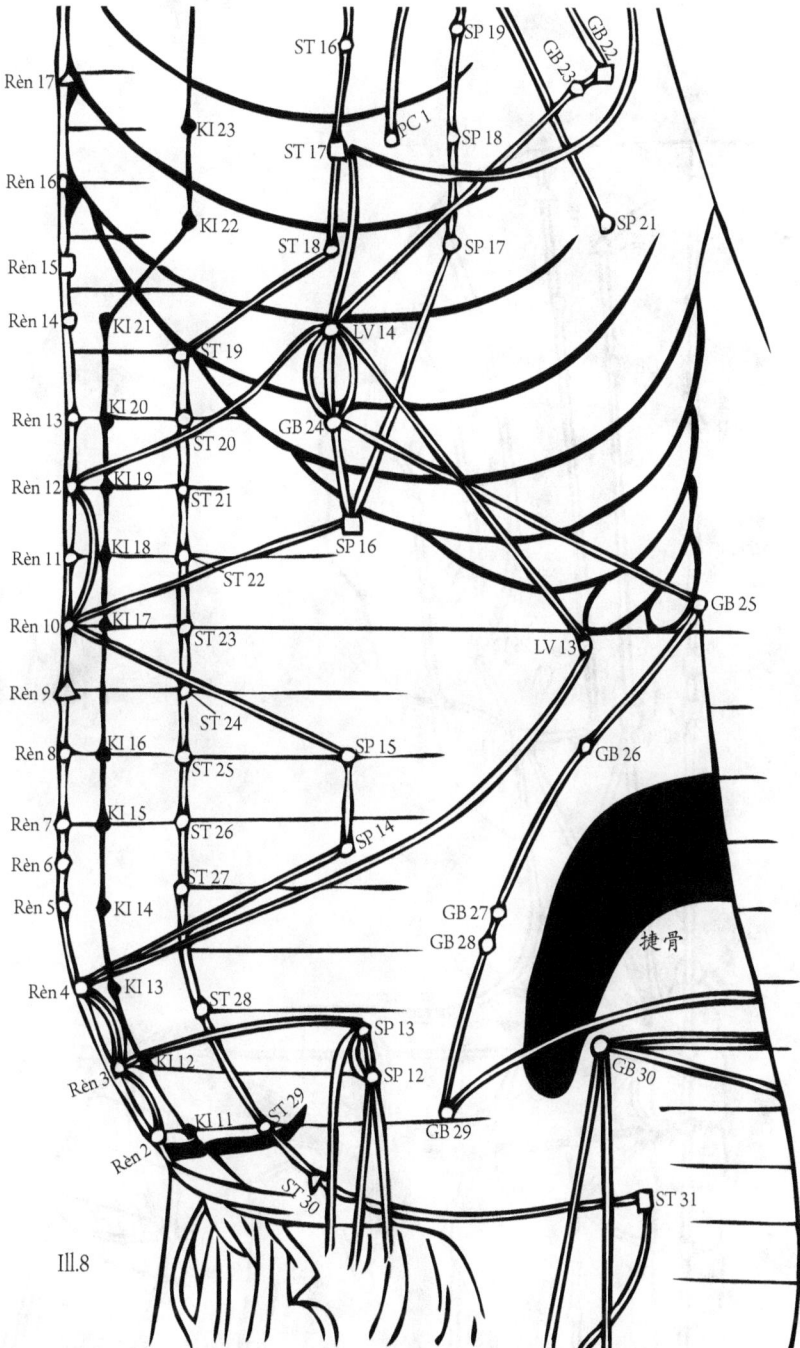

Ill.8

捷骨

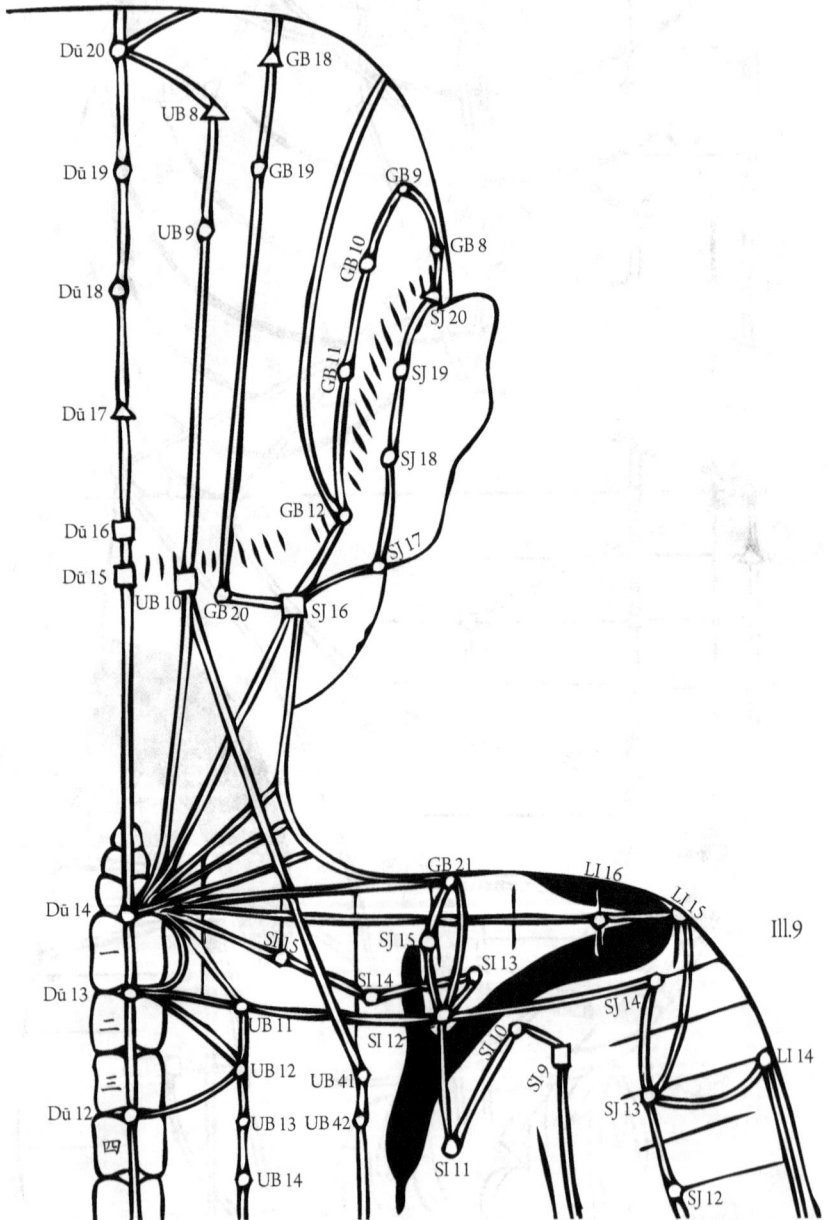

Ill.9

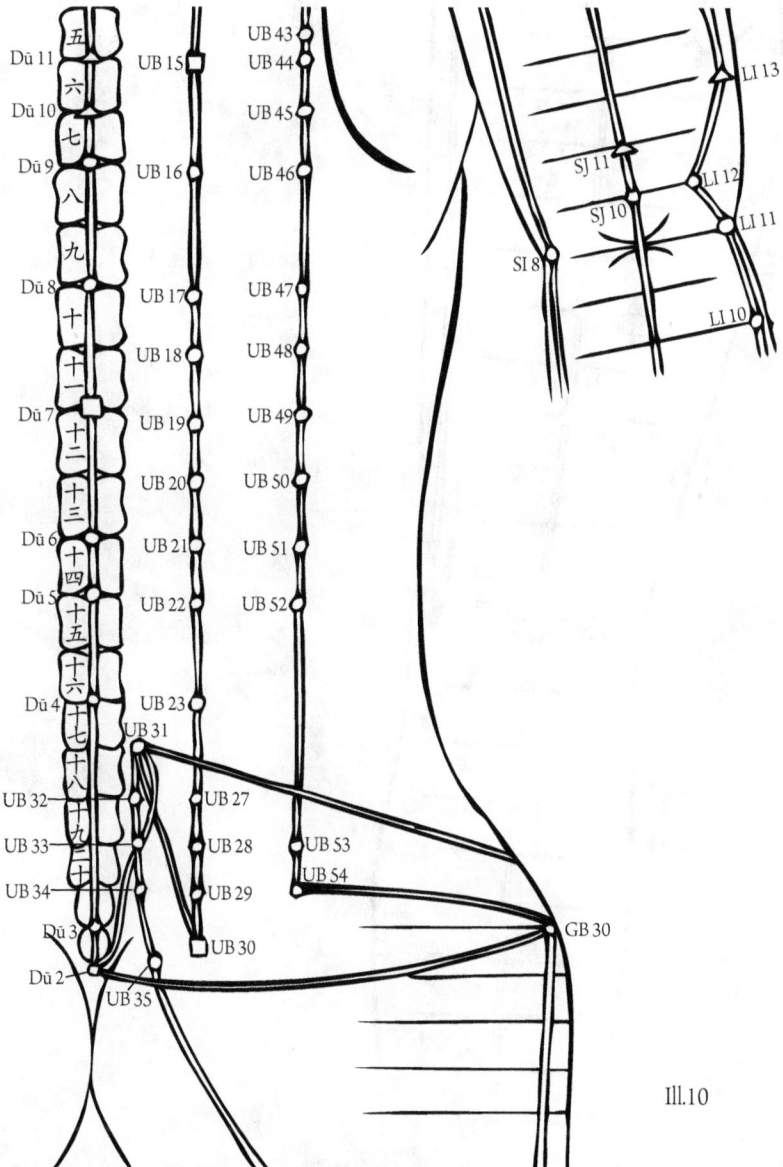

Ill.10

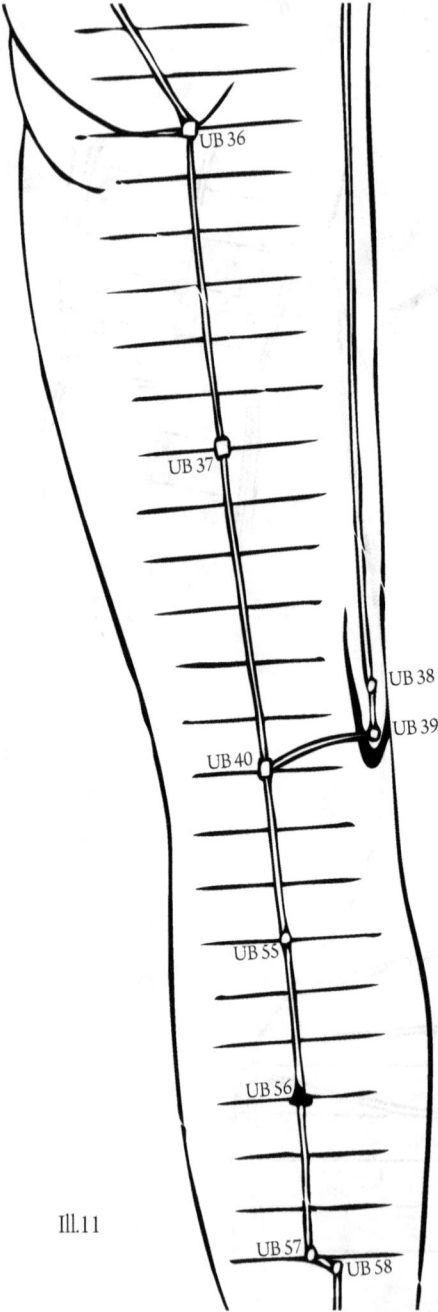

Ill.11

《靈樞·骨度第十四》
Líng Shū • Gǔ Dù (Bone Measurement), Chapter 14

黃帝問於伯高曰：脈度言經脈之長短，何以立之？伯高曰：
先度其骨節之大小、廣狹、長短，而脈度定矣。

Huángdì asked Bógāo: Vessel Measurement (*Mài Dù*)[1] speaks of the length of the channel-vessels; how is this established?

Bógāo said: First the size, the width, and the length of the bones and joints are measured, and then the vessel measurements are determined.

黃帝曰：願聞眾人之度。人長七尺五寸者，其骨節之大小長
短各幾何？伯高曰：頭之大骨圍，二尺六寸，胸圍四尺五
寸。腰圍四尺二寸。髮所覆者顱至項，尺二寸。髮以下至
頤，長一尺；君子終折。

Huángdì said: I want to hear the measurements of the average person. A human is 7.5 chǐ tall.[2] What is the size and length of each of his bone segments?

Bógāo said:
The circumference of the great bone of the head [the skull] is 2.6 chǐ.
The circumference of the chest is 4.5 chǐ.
The circumference of the waist is 4.2 chǐ.
Where the hair covers the skull to the nape is 1.2 chǐ.[3]
The length from below the hair to the chin is 1 chǐ.[4]

---

1. *Mài Dù* is the name of *Líng Shū*, Chapter 17; or this may instead refer to another ancient document.
2. One chǐ equals ten cùn, so 7.5 chǐ equals equals 75 cùn. Use this to convert chǐ to cùn, if desired, throughout this chapter.
3. In modern English, this would be the distance from the anterior hairline to the posterior hairline.
4. In modern English, this would be the distance from the anterior hairline to the lower edge of the mandible. *Yí* 頤, translated here as *chin*, is lateral to and

A superior person consults and corrects.[5]

結喉以下至缺盆中，長四寸。缺盆以下至髑骬，長九寸，過
則肺大，不滿則肺小。髑骬以下至天樞，長八寸，過則胃
大，不及則胃小。天樞以下至橫骨，長六寸半，過則迴腸廣
長，不滿則狹短。橫骨，長六寸半。橫骨上廉以下至內輔之
上廉，長一尺八寸。內輔之上廉以下至下廉，長三寸半。內
輔下廉，下至內踝，長一尺三寸。內踝以下至地，長三寸。
膝膕以下至跗屬，長一尺六寸。跗屬以下至地，長三寸。故
骨圍大則太過，小則不及。

The length from the laryngeal prominence down to the center [point between]
quē pén[6] is 4 cùn.

The length from quē pén down to hé yú[7] is 9 cùn. If it goes past this, the lungs
are large; if it does not fill this, the lungs are small.

The length from hé yú down to tiān shū[8] is 8 cùn. If it goes past this, the stomach is large; if it does not reach this, the stomach is small.

The length from tiān shū down to héng gŭ[9] is 6.5 cùn. If it goes past this, the
circling intestine (*huí cháng*) is wide and long; if it does not fill this, it is narrow
and short.

The length [width] of héng gŭ is 6.5 cùn.

The length from the upper aspect of héng gŭ down to the upper aspect of the
inner bumper bones[10] is 1.8 chǐ.

---

below the corners of the mouth, anterior to the cheeks; it is the region of Dà
Yíng (ST 5).

5. Meaning, a superior person adapts these measurements for different bodies.
This reading is based on various commentaries.

6. *Quē pén* 缺盆: the 'empty basin.' This is the supraclavicular fossa, from the
clavicle to the scapular spine; or the name of ST 12.

7. *Hé yú* 髑骬: The xiphoid process. (Huá Shòu said it means the junction of
the bones - the subcostal angle).

8. *Tiān shū* 天樞: The name of ST 25. However, this chapter does not focus on
points. The meaning (heaven's pivot) more likely refers to the dividing point
between heaven (the upper body) and earth (the lower body) at the waist.

9. *Héng gŭ* 橫骨 means the horizontal bone. It refers to the pubic bone and is
also the name of KI 11.

10. *Nèi fŭ* 內輔 inner bumper bones: Bumper bones indicates the bones on

The length from the upper aspect of the inner bumper bones down to its lower aspect is 3.5 cùn.

The length from the lower aspect of the inner bumper bones down to the inner malleolus is 1.3 chǐ.

The length from the inner malleolus down to the ground is 3 cùn.

The length from the back of the knee (*xī guó*, popliteal fossa) down to fū shǔ[11] is 1.6 chǐ.

The length from fū shǔ down to the ground is 3 cùn.

Thus, when the circumference of a bone is larger, it is goes beyond [the standard length]; when smaller, it fails to reach [the standard length].

角以下至柱骨，長一尺。行腋中不見者，長四寸。腋以下至季脅，長一尺二寸。季脅以下至髀樞，長六寸。髀樞以下至膝中，長一尺九寸。膝以下至外踝，長一尺六寸。外踝以下至京骨，長三寸。京骨以下至地，長一寸。

The length from the corner [of the forehead] down to the pillar bone[12] is 1 chǐ.

The length moving to the unseen center of the axilla[13] is 4 cùn.

The length from the axilla down to the free ribs is 1.2 chǐ.

The length from the free ribs down to the hip pivot[14] is 6 cùn.

The length from the hip pivot down to the center of the knee is 1.9 chǐ.

The length from the knee down to the outer malleolus is 1.6 chǐ.

---

both sides of the knees. On the inside is the *nèi fǔ* 內輔 (the bony protrusion of the medial condyle of the femur and the medial condyle of the tibia combined) and on the outside is the *wài fǔ* 外輔 (the bony protrusion of the lateral condyle of the femur and the lateral condyle of the tibia combined). The original meaning of *fǔ* 輔 was the protective bars on both sides of a cart, hence the image of the protrusion on both sides of the knee joint.

11. *Fū shǔ* 跗屬: This probably means the superior border of tuberosity of calcaneus.

12. *Zhù gǔ* 柱骨 (pillar bone): This refers to the cervical vertebrae; sometimes only C_7, sometimes C_4, C_5, and C_6, and sometimes even the clavicle. Here, commentators tend to feel it means the protruding bone at the base of the neck, usually C_7.

13. Zhāng Jièbīn commented that this sentence means the length from the pillar bone to the unseen center of the axilla.

14. *Bì shū* 髀樞 (hip pivot): The hip joint; or the upper outer part of the hip; or the great trochanter or acetabulum; or the name of GB 30.

The length from the outer malleolus down to jīng gŭ[15] is 3 cùn.
The length from jīng gŭ down to the ground is 1 cùn.

耳後當完骨者，廣九寸。耳前當耳門者，廣一尺三寸。兩顴
之間，相去七寸。兩乳之間，廣九寸半。兩髀之間，廣六寸
半。

The width behind the ears right at wán gŭ[16] is 9 cùn.
The width in front of the ears right at ěr mén[17] is 1.3 chǐ.
The cheekbones[18] are 7 cùn from each other.
The width between the nipples is 9.5 cùn.
The width between the hips is 6.5 cùn.[19]

足長一尺二寸，廣四寸半。肩至肘，長一尺七寸。肘至腕，
長一尺二寸半。腕至中指本節，長四寸。本節至其末，長四
寸半。

A foot is 1.2 chǐ long and 4.5 cùn wide.
The length from the shoulder to the elbow is 1.7 chǐ.
The length from the elbow to the wrist is 1.25 chǐ.
The length from the wrist to the base joint of the middle finger is 4 cùn.
The length from the base joint to the end [of the middle finger] is 4.5 cùn.

項髮以下至背骨，長二寸半。膂骨以下至尾骶，二十一節，
長三尺。上節長一寸四分分之一，奇分在下，故上七節至于
膂骨，九寸八分分之七。此眾人骨之度也，所以立經脈之長
短也。

---

15. *Jīng gŭ* 京骨: The base of the fifth metatarsal bone, or the name of UB 64.
16. *Wán gŭ* 完骨: The mastoid process or the name of GB 12.
17. *Ěr mén* 耳門: The tragus or the name of SJ 21.
18. *Quán* 顴 (cheekbone): The lateral cheekbones, the high bone lateral to and below the eyelids.
19. Zhāng Jièbīn commented that this means the distance between the inner thighs. Above, the text said, "The length of *héng gŭ* is 6.5 cùn." This would be in agreement.

The length from the hair at the nape down to the back bone[20] is 2.5 cùn.[21]
The length of the 21 segments from lǚ gǔ[22] down to the sacrum-coccyx (wěi dǐ) is 3 chǐ.

The upper segments[23] are 1.41 cùn long [height] and are not paired with those below, thus the length of the upper 7 segments down to lǚ gǔ is 9.87 cùn. These are the measurements of the bones for the average person; it is what is used to establish the length of the channel-vessels.

是故視其經脈之在於身也，其見浮而堅，其見明而大者，多血，細而沉者，多氣也。

Therefore one inspects the channel-vessels in the person's body; those that appear to be floating and solid, or appear to be bright and large have copious blood;[24] those that are fine and deep have copious qì.

---

20. *Tài Sù* and *Jiǎ Yǐ Jīng* both have lǚ gǔ 膂骨 here rather than bèi gǔ 背骨 (back bone).
21. *Tài Sù* and *Jiǎ Yǐ Jīng* both have 3.5 cùn rather than 2.5 cùn.
22. *Lǚ gǔ* 膂骨: The spinous process of the first thoracic vertebra, or the spine as a whole. Here, it seems to mean T_1.
23. The *upper segments* refers to the cervical vertebrae.
24. This should refer to the luò vessels.

《靈樞・背腧第五十一》
Líng Shū • Bèi Shù (The Back Shù Points), Chapter 51

黃帝問於岐伯曰：願聞五臟之腧，出於背者。

Huángdì asked Qí Bó: I would like to hear about the *shù* points of the five *zàng*-organs, which emerge on the back.

岐伯曰：背中大腧，在杼骨之端，肺腧在三焦之間，心腧在五焦之間，膈腧在七焦之間，肝腧在九焦之間，脾腧在十一焦之間，腎腧在十四焦之間。

Qí Bó said: The great *shù* points on the back are located at the ends of the shuttle bones [vertebrae].
The lung *shù* (UB 13) is located in the space of the third vertebra[25] [T_3].
The heart *shù* (UB 15) is located in the space of the fifth vertebra [T_5].
The diaphragm *shù* (UB 17) is located in the space of the seventh vertebra [T_7].
The liver *shù* (UB 18) is located in the space of the ninth vertebra [T_9].
The spleen *shù* (UB 20) is located in the space of the eleventh vertebra [T_{11}].
The kidney *shù* (UB 23) is located in the space of the fourteenth vertebra [L_2].[26]

皆挾脊相去三寸所，則欲得而驗之，按其處，應在中而痛解，乃其輸也。

All of them embrace the spine and are located 3 cùn from each other.[27] When you want to locate and examine them, press on the site. If it responds within, the pain will resolve and it is [the patient's] *shù* point.[28]

---

25. The text has *jiāo* 焦 (burner) where it is translated as *zhuī* 椎 (vertebra). Wáng Bīng's 王冰 notes, *Tài Sù* 《太素》, and *Jiǎ Yǐ Jīng* 《甲乙經》 all use *zhuī* 椎 (vertebra) in the parallel passage.
26. Note that the *shù* points of the yáng organs are never mentioned.
27. They are 1.5 cùn to each side of the spine, which makes them 3 cùn from each other.
28. Note the importance of palpation in locating these points.

灸之則可，刺之則不可。氣盛則瀉之，虛則補之。以火補者，毋吹其火，須自滅也；以火瀉之，疾吹其火，傳其艾，須其火滅也。

You can apply moxibustion to them but you cannot prick them.[29] When qì is exuberant, drain it; when it is deficient, supplement it. To use fire [moxibustion] to supplement, do not blow on the fire; you must let it extinguish itself. To use fire to drain, quickly blow on the fire to spread [radiate] the mugwort [qì], and you must extinguish the fire.[30]

---

29. The back *shù* points were originally contraindicated for pricking. Perhaps before angle and depth were worked out, there were accidents with needling. However, moxibustion was and still is favored. Even today, treatment of the back *shù* points commonly relies on moxibustion more than some of the other points.

30. This last line is somewhat problematic. The language is not very clear. Historically, different commentators have interpreted it a little differently. It seems that the main idea is this: To supplement, let the mugwort fire burn down slowly and extinguish itself. In this way, the yáng of the moxa can go into the point. To drain, blow on the burning cone. This makes a more intense heat which can radiate the evil outward and away. However, the mugwort fire gets extinguished before the fire reaches the skin, so nothing enters the point.

《素問·血氣形志篇第二十四》 (節選)

Sù Wèn· Xuè Qì Xíng Zhì Piān (Plain Questions·Qì and Blood [of the Channels] and Body and Mind) Chapter 24 (Excerpted)

欲知背俞，先度其兩乳間，中折之。更以他草度，去半已，
即以兩隅相拄也。

If one wants to know [the location of] the back transport points, first measure [the distance between] the nipples [with a piece of straw] and fold it in the center. Alter another piece of straw, measuring, and once half [of the length of straw] is removed, use the two corners to support each other.

乃舉以度其背，令其一隅居上，齊脊大椎，兩隅在下，當其
下隅者，肺之俞也。

Then hold the measuring [straw] on the back. Make the upper corner even with Dà Zhuī (Dū 14) on the spine. The two lower corners will be at the back transport point of the lungs (UB 13).

復下一度，心之俞也。

Repeat one time below for the back transport point of the heart (UB 15).

復下一度，左角，肝之俞也；右角，脾之俞也；

111

Repeat one[31] time below for the back transport point of the liver (UB 18) at the left[32] corner and the spleen (UB 20) at the right[33] corner.

復下一度，腎之俞也。

Repeat one time below for the back transport point of the kidneys (UB 23).

是謂五臟之俞。灸刺之度也。

These are [the location of] the back transport points of the fiver viscera. It is the standard for [locating] acupuncture [points].

---

31. The straw measuring device is moved downward so that the upper corner of it is on the center of the spine at the same level as the transport point that was just located. The next back transport point is supposed to be at the two bottom corners of the triangle. This measurement is moved downward in this way three times for a total of four levels. Each time the measurement is repeated, it should be approximately the distance of two or three vertebrae (the distance between Du 14 and UB 13; the distance between UB 13 and UB 15). In reality, this method will not bring us to the same point location we use today. It will also differ from *Líng Shū • Bèi Shù* 《靈樞· 背腧第五十一 》(The Back Shù Points), Chapter 51. The problem is that there are different number of vertebrae between different back transport points and the vertebrae are not all the same size.

32. According to *Tài Sù* 《太素 》(Grand Simplicity of the Yellow Emperor's Inner Classic) by Yáng Shàngshàn 楊上善 (*Suí* 隋 dynasty) and *Yī Xīn Fāng* 《醫心方 》(Jp: *Ishinpo*) by Tamba Yasuyori (984), this should say the right corner.

33. The above-mentioned texts also note that this should say the left corner. This location of the liver transport (UB 18) and the spleen transport (UB 20) are different than what we use today since UB 20 and UB 18 are not now considered to be at the same level. This also differs from *Líng Shū • Bèi Shù* 《靈樞· 背腧第五十一 》(The Back Shù Points), Chapter 51.

Text Index

People Index

Points Index

Dà Zhuī	(Dū 14)	38, 60–85, 111	Xìn Huì	(Dū 22)		32
Yǎ Mén	(Dū 15)	31	Shéng Tíng	(Dū 24)		32
Fēng Fǔ	(Dū 16)	31	Sù Liáo	(Dū 25)		31
Nǎo Hù	(Dū 17)	32				

General Index

The Chinese Medicine Database

www.cm-db.com

The Chinese Medicine Database has been organized around one central principle -- translation of Classical Asian texts, and dissemination of that information.

There are thousands of Asian medicine texts that have never been translated. We have compiled a small list on our website of the ones that we have found, but we believe that there are tens of thousands of documents that span from the *Hàn* Dynasty to pre-Republican times. Most of these documents will never be read by people in the West, simply because of lack of translation.

We have created a vehicle, that allows interested practitioners, students, institutions, and scholars to help support and fund the translation of these documents, and then mine and synthesize the data that is gained from these texts.

The Database contains:

Monographs on:
690 Single Herbs
1510 Formulas
Mayway's Patents
ITM's Formulations
Golden Flowers Formulations
Classical Pearls Formulations by Heiner Fruehauf
OBGYN Modifications to Formulas
Single Points: the 361 Regular Points
Time Line of the History of Chinese Medicine

Beer Hall Lecture Series:
Watch videos from our monthly Beer Hall lecture series with guest speakers such as: Arnaud Versluys, Subhuti Dharmananda, Jason Robertson, Craig Mitchell, Michael Max, Lorraine Wilcox, and Ed Neal.

CEU/ PDA/ Livestreaming Lectures:
We now have a stand alone video system which allows people to watch lectures without being a subscriber. These lectures feature top quality lecturers speaking on classical Chinese medicine and medicinals. This can be found at: http://cm-db.com/xstreaming.php

Play STORT:

Play our free online game STORT where you can learn Chinese while having a bit of fun (www.cm-db.com/stort).

A Chinese-English dictionary:

Containing over 105,000 terms, including the Eastland and the WHO term sets.

Our Translation Tools:

A pop-up translation system using the terminology in our books, as well as our Chinese-English dictionary system. This allows the user to translate their own documents out of Chinese.

Translations:

Shāng Hán Lái Sū Jí	傷寒來蘇集	Renewal of Treatise on Cold Damage
Qí Jīng Bā Mài Kǎo	奇經八脈考	Explanation of the Eight Vessels of the Marvellous Meridians
Shāng Hán Míng Lǐ Lùn	傷寒明理論	Treatise on Enlightening the Principles of Cold Damage
Wú Jū Tōng Yī Àn	吳鞠通医案	Case Studies of Wú Jūtōng
The Nàn Jīng	難經	The Classic of Difficulties
The Zàng Fǔ Biāo Běn Hán Rè Xū Shí Yòng Yào Shì	臟腑標本寒熱虛實用藥式	Viscera and Bowels, Tip and Root, Cold and Heat, Vacuity and Repletion Model for Using Medicinals
Wēn Rè Lún	温熱論	Treatise on Warm Heat Disease
Shāng Hán Shé Jiàn	傷寒舌鑒	Tongue Mirror of Cold Damage
Xǔ Shì Yī Àn	許氏醫案	Case Histories of Master Xǔ
Fǔ Xíng Jué Zāng Fǔ Yòng Yào Fǎ Yào	輔行決臟腑用藥法要	Secret Instructions for Assisting the Body: Essential Methods for the Application of Drugs to the Viscera & Bowels
Biāo Yōu Fù	標幽賦	Indicating the Obscure
Liú Juān Zǐ Guǐ Yí Fāng	劉涓子鬼遺方	Liu Juanzi's Formulas Inherited from Ghosts
Shèn Jí Chú Yán	慎疾芻言	Precautions in Illness: My Humble Thoughts
Yào Zhèng Jì Yí	藥症忌宜	Medicinals & Patterns Contraindications & Appropriate [Choices]
Fù Kē Wèn Dá	婦科問答	Questions and Answers in Gynecology
Nèi Jīng Zhī Yào	内經知要	Essential Knowledge from the Nèijīng

| Běn Cǎo Bèi Yào | 本草備要 | The Essential Completion of Traditional Materia Medica |
| Bǎi Zhèng Fù (Jù Yīng) | 百症賦《聚英》 | Ode of the Hundred Diseases from The Great Compendium of Acupuncture-Moxibustion |

Benefits:

Subscribers to the Database receive a 10% discount on our published books when they are in pre-release.

Published Books:

2008 Bèi Jí Qiān Jīn Yào Fāng 備急千金要方:
Essential Prescriptions Worth a Thousand Gold Pieces For Emergencies. vol. 2-4
by Sūn Sīmiǎo 孫思邈
Translated by Sabine Wilms.
ISBN 978-0-9799552-0-4
Permanently Out of Print

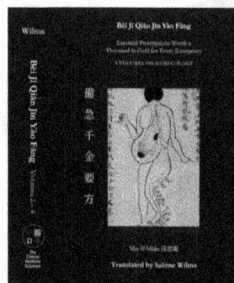

2010 Zhēn Jiǔ Dà Chéng 針灸大成:
The Great Compendium of Acupuncture & Moxibustion vol. I
by Yáng Jìzhōu 楊繼洲
Translated by Sabine Wilms.
ISBN 978-0-9799552-2-8

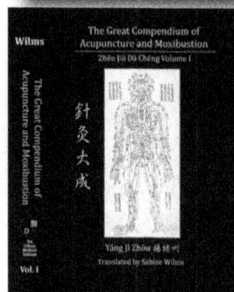

2010 Zhēn Jiǔ Dà Chéng 針灸大成:
The Great Compendium of Acupuncture & Moxibustion vol. V
by Yáng Jìzhōu 楊繼洲
Translated by Lorraine Wilcox.
ISBN 978-0-9799552-4-2

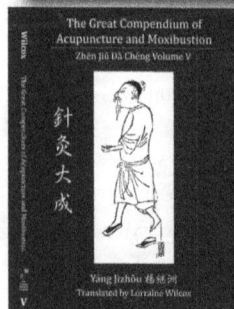

2010 Jīn Guì Fāng Gē Kuò 金匱方歌括:
Formulas from the Golden Cabinet with Songs vol. I - III
by Chén Xiūyuán 陳修園
Translated by Sabine Wilms.
ISBN 978-0-9799552-5-9

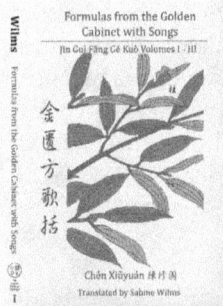

2011 Zhēn Jiǔ Dà Chéng 針灸大成:
The Great Compendium of Acupuncture & Moxibustion
vol. VIII
by Yáng Jìzhōu 楊繼洲
Translated by Yue Lu.
ISBN 978-0-9799552-7-3

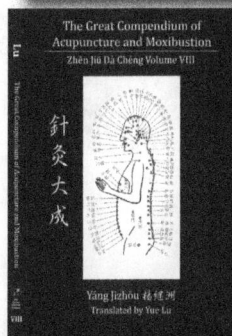

2011 Zhēn Jiǔ Dà Chéng 針灸大成:
The Great Compendium of Acupuncture & Moxibustion
vol. IX
by Yáng Jìzhōu 楊繼洲
Translated by Lorraine Wilcox.
ISBN 978-0-9799552-6-6

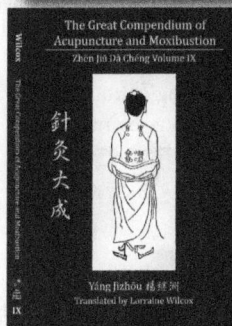

2012 Raising the Dead and Returning Life: Emergency
Medicine of the Qīng Dynasty
by Bào Xiāng'áo 鮑相璈
Translated by Lorraine Wilcox.
ISBN 978-0-9799552-3-5

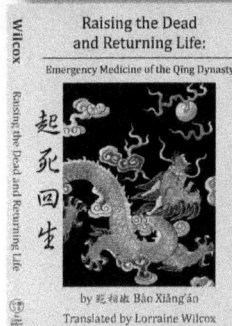

2014 Zhēn Jiǔ Zī Shēng Jīng 針灸資生經:
The Classic of Supporting Life with Acupuncture and
Moxibustion Vol. I-III
by Wáng Zhízhōng 王執中
Translated by Yue Lu.
ISBN 978-0-9799552-1-1

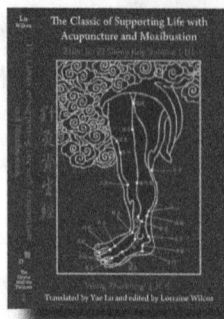

2014 Jīn Guì Fāng Gē Kuò 金匱方歌括:
Formulas from the Golden Cabinet with Songs
vol. IV - VI
by Chén Xiūyuán 陳修園
Translated by Eran Even.
ISBN 978-0-9799552-8-0

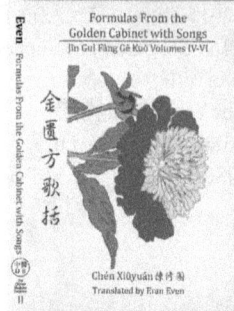

2015 Zhēn Jiǔ Zī Shēng Jīng 針灸資生經:
The Classic of Supporting Life with Acupuncture and
Moxibustion Vol. IV-VII
by Wáng Zhízhōng 王執中
Translated by Yue Lu.
ISBN 978-0-9799552-9-7

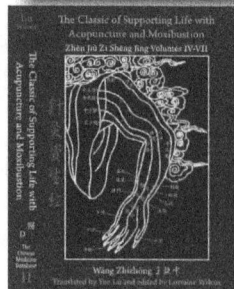

2015 Nǚ Yī Zá Yán 女醫雜言:
Miscellaneous Records of a Female Doctor
by Tán Yǔnxián 談允賢
Translated by Lorraine Wilcox.
ISBN 978-0-9906029-0-3

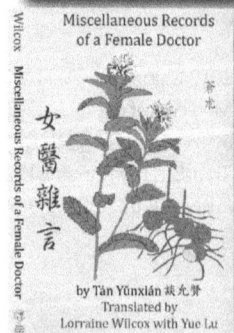

2016 Nǔ Kē Cuō Yào 女科撮要:
Outline of Female Medicine
by Xuē Jǐ 薛己
Translated by Lorraine Wilcox.
ISBN 978-0-9906029-1-0

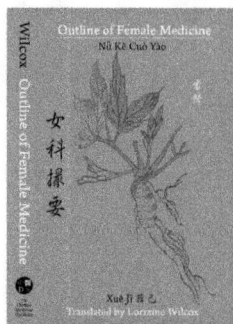

2016 Shén Nóng Běn Cǎo Jīng Dú 神農本草經讀:
Reading of the Divine Farmer's Classic of Materia Medica
by Chén Xiūyuán 陳修園
Translated by Corinna Theisinger.
ISBN 978-0-9906029-2-7

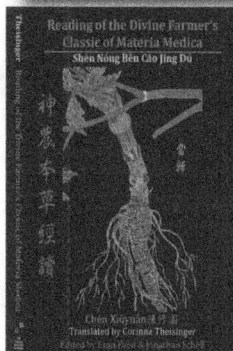

2017 Zhèng Tǐ Lèi Yào 正體類要:
Categorized Essentials of Repairing the Body
by Xuē Jǐ 薛己
Translated by Lorraine Wilcox.
ISBN 978-0-9906029-3-4

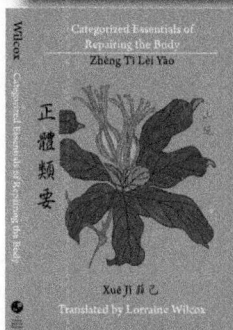

2018 Zhù Jiě Shāng Hán Lùn 注解傷寒論:
Commentary On The Discussion of Cold Damage With
Annotations
by Chéng Wújǐ 成無己
Translated by Jonathan Schell L.Ac..
ISBN 978-0-9906029-4-1

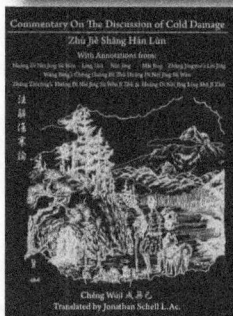

2018 Fukushō-Kiran 腹證奇覽:
Extraordinary Views of Abdominal Patterns
by Inaba Katsu Bunrei 稲葉克文禮
Translated by Jay Kageyama
ISBN: 978-0-9906029-5-8

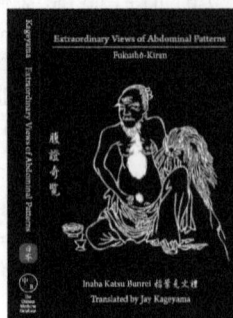